Hilary Thoms

# GCSE Health & Social Care

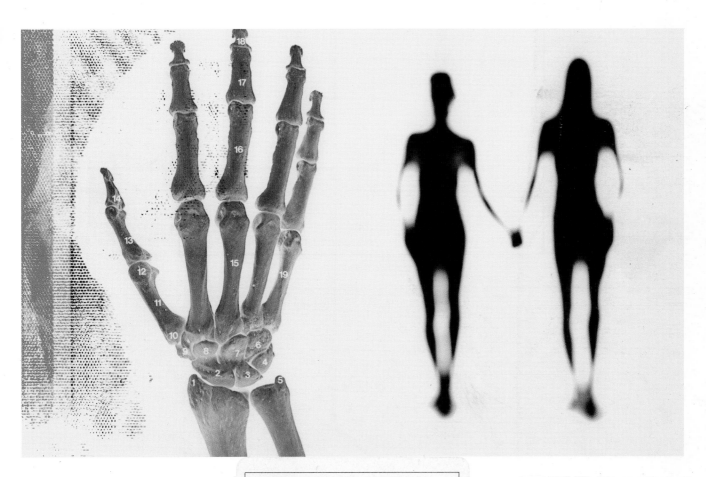

Orders: please contact Bookpoint Ltd, 130 Milton Park, Abingdon, Oxon OX14 4SB. Telephone: (44) 01235 827720, Fax: (44) 01235 400454. Lines are open from 9.00 - 6.00, Monday to Saturday, with a 24 hour message answering service.

*British Library Cataloguing in Publication Data*
A catalogue record for this title is available from The British Library

ISBN 0340 85782X

First published 2002

Impression number  10 9 8 7 6 5 4 3 2 1
Year                        2007 2006 2005 2004 2003 2002

Copyright © 2002 Hilary Thomson, Sylvia Aslangul, Caroline Holden

Cover photo from Getty Images

Typeset by Pantek Arts Ltd, Maidstone, Kent.
Printed in Italy for Hodder & Stoughton Educational, a division of Hodder Headline Plc, 338 Euston Road, London NW1 3BH.

# Contents

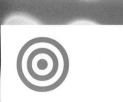

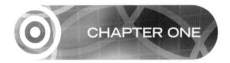
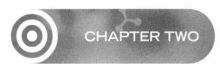

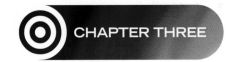
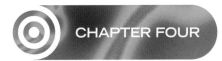

# Acknowledgements

Photo credits: Figure 2.22 Photofusion; Figure 2.34 Jacky Chapman; Figure 2.41 Sally Greenhill; Figure 2.42 Sally Greenhill; Figure 3.4 Paula Solloway; Figure 3.5 Dave Thompson; Figure 3.11 Emma Lee; Figure 3.12 Sally Greenhill; Figure 3.13 Action Plus;Figure 3.26 National Medical Slide Bank; Figure 3.29 getty Images; Figure 3.30 Getty Images; Figure 3.32 National Medical Slide Bank; Figure 3.33 Sally Greenhill; Figure 4.2(a) Sally Greenhill; Figure 4.2(b) Sally Greenhill; Figure 4.2(c) National Medical Slide Bank

Chapter 2: Figure 2.14 Tooting NHS Walk In Centre; Figures 2.14, 2.17, 2.46, London Borough of Sutton; Figures 2.22, 2.41, 2.42 Weekend Project Sutton; Table 2.6 Merton Sutton and Wandsworth Health Authority; Figure 2.23 Family Focus Sutton; Fig 2.28, Case Study 8, Sutton Carers Centre; Figure 3.30 Envok Language Services; Case studies of nurses, Sally Savageot, Joyce Bentley; Figure 2.36 London Borough of Merton; Figure 2.50 South West London Community Trust; Figure 2.53 Stroke Association.

Chapter 4: Figure 4.29 Foundation for the study of Infant Deaths (SFID) and thanks to nurses, doctors, staff, carers and patients for allowing me to use their experiences in this book.

Crown copyright is reproduced with the Permission of the Controller of HMSO and the Queen's Printer for Scotland.

Every effort has been made to trace the copyright holders of material reproduced in this book. Any rights omitted from the acknowledgements here or in the text will be added for subsequent printings following notice to the publisher.

# Learning to learn: a study skills guide

1

Students taking the Vocational GCSE in Health and Social Care will find that the course is designed with several purposes in mind. One is to enable students to gain knowledge, understanding and experience in the vocational area of health and social care. Another is to **learn how to learn** more effectively.

Most students will cope well with the demands this course makes upon them. Others may need to investigate new ways to manage difficulties they have always experienced, perhaps because of a condition such as dyslexia or a disability. There are also certain people, such as older students returning to study after a break from education, who may find they need extra study skills support.

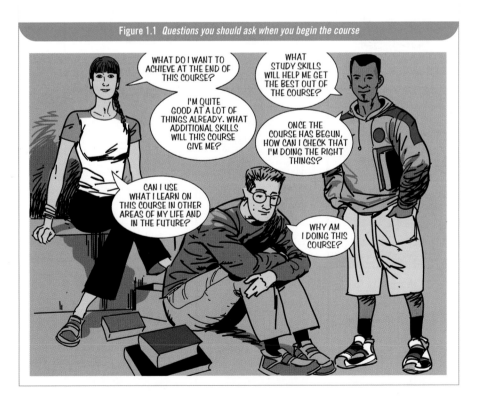

**Figure 1.1** *Questions you should ask when you begin the course*

For all of us, however, learning how to learn is **essential for success**. Students who take the following advice to heart will achieve the best results:

"Wise is she who knows when she does not know!"

This chapter has been written to help you become an independent learner, able to make your own decisions about how to approach coursework assignments, tests, work experience, future study and career choices.

As you begin the course, take time to ask yourself the questions illustrated in Figure 1.1. Discuss any issues they raise with your teachers, tutors and fellow students.

# CHAPTER CONTENT

This chapter covers:

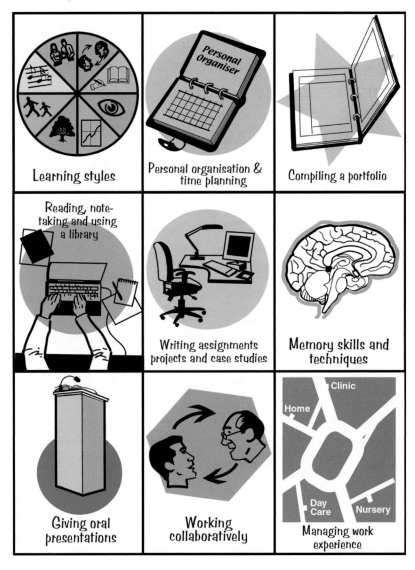

| | | |
|---|---|---|
| Learning styles | Personal organisation & time planning | Compiling a portfolio |
| Reading, note-taking and using a library | Writing assignments projects and case studies | Memory skills and techniques |
| Giving oral presentations | Working collaboratively | Managing work experience |

The chapter also offers support for the development of Key Skills. Key Skills are the general skills that can help you improve your own learning and performance. They are relevant to what you do in education, training, work and life in general. Students taking this course will also be working towards gaining a Key Skills qualification. This qualification recognises achievement in the six Key Skills Units of:

▶ Communication

▶ Application of Number

▶ Information Technology

▶ Working with Others

▶ Improving Own Learning and Performance

▶ Problem-solving

This chapter encourages you to focus upon **what** you are learning and **how** you are learning. It will therefore indicate opportunities for demonstrating the relevant aspects of each Key Skill. The chapter concludes with a glossary and a list of useful resources.

# LEARNING STYLES

All of us learn in different ways. We each have a combination of different types of intelligence. While some people may be good all-rounders who are able to learn, depending upon the task in hand, through a wide variety of methods, others may find it much easier to use just one or two **learning styles**. A learning style is a way of taking in and processing information. For example, some people are organised and analytical. They make lists of what they have to do and plan their time carefully. Others do things when they occur to them, sometimes on the spur of the moment, often prompted by ideas they have been thinking about for a while. While some people learn best by listening and discussing things, others need to 'see' information visually, in pictures, diagrams and colours.

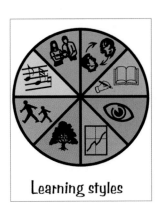

Learning styles

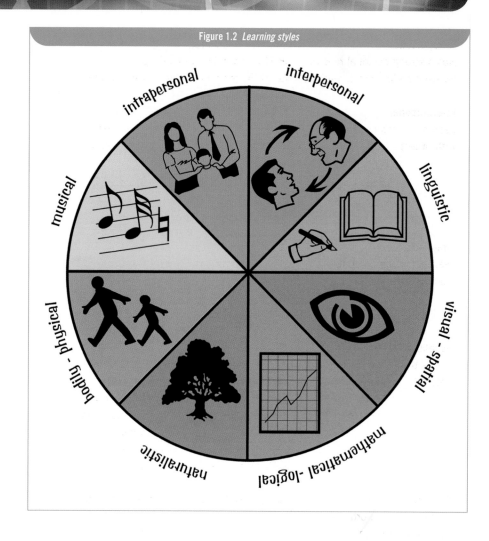

Figure 1.2 *Learning styles*

# Activity

1. What are your preferred learning styles? Use Figure 1.2 and Table 1.1 to think about the methods of working that suit you best. Make a note of these. You will need to keep these in mind as you read this chapter.

2. Are you an all-rounder (with no strong preference for any particular way of working), or do you find certain methods of working easier than others?

3. Use the Internet to find out more about learning styles. There are many good sites. Use a web browser such as Google at www.google.com and type in *learning styles*. Find and try out one or two of the interesting interactive online 'learning styles' tests.

**Intrapersonal**
Has a strong personal reason for wanting to learn something.

- Is self-motivated.
- Understands own feelings.
- Motivated by a strong sense of values.

**Interpersonal**
Learns through communication with others

- Is a good listener and/or speaker.
- Can see an issue from different perspectives.
- Is able to understand other people's behaviour and ideas.
- Can build relationships with others.
- Enjoys teamwork and discussion.
- Is a good organiser.

**Linguistic**
Learns through listening, reading, writing and discussion.

- Enjoys discussions.
- Is a good communicator.
- May find mnemonics useful.
- May find it helpful to tape-record lessons/lectures to listen to again.

**Visual/spatial**
Learns through visualising material.

- Tends to think in 'pictures'.
- Can make three-dimensional objects.
- Enjoys using multimedia.
- Prefers to use colour, pictures, charts, maps, graphs and mind-maps in written work.
- Prefers to read books with plenty of illustrations and visual material.
- Learns through seeing and doing.

**Mathematical/logical**
Uses sequences, order and logic to learn things.

- Can see the relationship between objects and ideas.
- Can find solutions to problems.
- Enjoys experiments.
- Can think conceptually and is curious about the world.

**Naturalistic**
Learns through a 'hands-on' approach.

- Needs to do things actively, with a sense of exploration.
- Enjoys experiments.
- Feels in tune with the natural environment.
- Concerned about environmental issues.

**Bodily/physical/kinaesthetic**
Learns through touch, movement and physical exercise.

- Is skilful with objects.
- Learns by doing.
- May need to take frequent short breaks when studying.
- Chewing gum/listening to music when studying may aid concentration.

**Musical**
Rhythm and music may aid memory and concentration when studying something.

- Is sensitive to the effect of music on mood.
- Uses musical ability/sense of rhythm to remember things (e.g. musical jingles).
- Enjoys listening to music when studying.

*Table 1.1 Learning styles*

People working in health and social care need good interpersonal and intrapersonal skills. It would not be surprising if students who chose to study this course felt they were strong in these areas or wanted to develop these particular skills. However, while we may learn best through channels that work for us, there is nothing to stop us from exploring new ways to learn. The rest of this chapter contains many ideas for studying effectively and for developing competence in the wide range of academic and vocational skills required from students taking the Vocational GCSE in Health and Social Care.

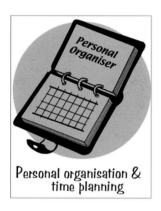

Personal organisation & time planning

# PERSONAL ORGANISATION AND TIME PLANNING

Virtually any activity (washing dishes, tidying your room, staring at the wall, fetching just *one more* small snack) can seem preferable to working on an assignment or settling down to revision. However, when work is postponed regularly, deadlines and examination dates can increase feelings of disorganisation and panic and can trigger a 'flight' response. It can become tempting to produce the minimum work possible, or even to abandon assignments com-

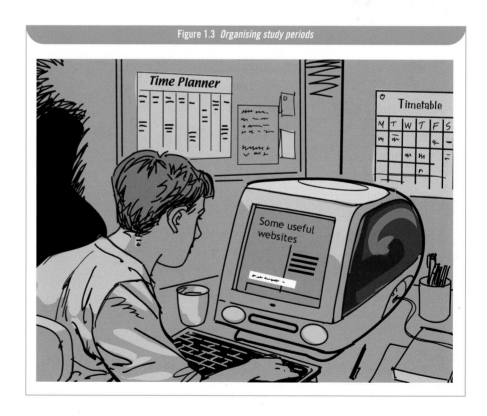

Figure 1.3 *Organising study periods*

pletely. Excuses have to be invented, deadlines renegotiated, further assignments become due before the last ones are completed and, before long, the course begins to feel overwhelming and unmanageable.

Of course, people can have very good reasons for finding their workload difficult to manage: child care or other family responsibilities; the need to earn money through part-time work and unexpected trauma or illness, can all increase the pressure on students. However, if you are generally enjoying your course and finding the work stimulating and interesting, you are likely to want to find a way of organising your time so that you can keep a balance between your work, your social life and your other interests and commitments.

## Planning time

There are only so many hours in a week. Although keeping rigidly to a **weekly planner** or timetable (such as the one shown in Table 1.2) will not always be easy or desirable, it should help you to focus on what free time you have in a week and which 'chunks' of it can be used for coursework and revision.

# Activity

Photocopy and enlarge the planner on page 8 or draw up your own.

Now mark on it:

▶ your college or school timetabled commitments, i.e. your lectures and lessons
▶ any paid work, housework or child care/family commitments
▶ travel times
▶ times you normally spend with friends/sports activities/other leisure pursuits
▶ any 'unmissable' T.V. programmes (not too many!).

What 'chunks' of time have you left for studying?

▶ In the day?
▶ In the evening?
▶ At weekends?

Table 1.2 *Weekly planner*

| | MONDAY | TUESDAY | WEDNESDAY | THURSDAY | FRIDAY | SATURDAY | SUNDAY |
|---|---|---|---|---|---|---|---|
| | Who can help? | Who can help? | Who can help? | Who can help? | Who can help? | Who can help? | Who can help? |
| | Best time to study? | Best time to study? | Best time to study? | Best time to study? | Best time to study? | Best time to study? | Best time to study? |
| morning | morning | morning | morning | morning | morning | morning | morning |
| afternoon | afternoon | afternoon | afternoon | afternoon | afternoon | afternoon | afternoon |
| evening | evening | evening | evening | evening | evening | evening | evening |

Every day is different, so note down when the best time for study will be each day. Will there be anyone who can help you with the work if you have problems? Note down times when parents/teachers/work-shops/homework or study skills clubs are available. Don't forget that the half-term or end of term holidays can be a good time to catch up on assignments and revision. Remember to include these in your long-term calculations. However, having completed your planner, will you need to readjust any commitments to give you enough time to complete coursework? How important will it be for you to spend some time studying in the day as well as in the evening?

To enable you to plan ahead to complete work on time, it will also be useful to keep a **diary** or **academic year planner** at hand to note down, for **all** your GCSE subjects, coursework deadlines, examination dates and dates of visits or work experience.

---

**Remember**, some people can happily juggle an enormous number of different commitments and activities in their lives. They thrive on the variety and stimulation of so much to do. Others prefer a slower pace, with fewer commitments and more time to concentrate upon each one. How you **find** and **manage** the time you need to complete the course successfully will mean thinking about what conditions **you** need for learning.

---

# Motivation during study periods

It is important to find a place where you can work without inter-ruptions and distractions. Even if you have the luxury of a room and a desk of your own at home, you will probably need to con-sider using your school, college or public library for some study periods. Settling down to a period of study is easier if you:

▶ remove all distractions of hunger, noise, cold, and sociable friends!

▶ try not to study if you are feeling angry or upset

▶ keep a pad of paper or a jotter next to you as you work – when ideas occur to you, you can note them down before you forget them

▶ give yourself realistic targets and decide before you start how long you will study for. Try not to work for more than an hour without a short break. Reward yourself for completing what you planned to do

- try to give yourself a variety of activities to work on
- take regular but short breaks
- have the phone number of someone else from your class or group handy in case you need to discuss the best way to go about a task or check what you need to do
- have a drink to hand (water is best)
- if you enjoy listening to music while you work, research seems to show that quieter, instrumental music (modern or classical) can aid concentration. Unsurprisingly, loud, percussive music appears to have the opposite effect!

# COMPILING A PORTFOLIO

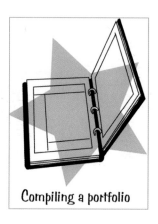

Compiling a portfolio

A **portfolio** is a collection of the different types of evidence that can be used to show successful completion of the course. Examples of evidence include:

- completed **assignments**, **projects** or **case studies**, including **action plans** and **evaluations**. These can be handwritten or word-processed, although work in the form of video recordings, audio-tape recordings, photographs, logbooks and diaries may also be acceptable where they contain evidence of the practical demonstration of skills. Check with your teacher or tutor.
- past **records of achievement**, **qualifications**, **work experience** or other evidence of **prior learning**.
- samples of relevant class or lecture **notes**, **lists**, **personal reading records** or **copies of letters** written (perhaps regarding work experience, to request information or advice, or related to job or further education applications).

## Equipment and materials

It will be worthwhile taking advantage of any cheap stationery offers at high street stores and equipping yourself with:

- at least **five large A4 lever arch files** and sets of **extra wide file dividers** (or large A4 box files). One of these files will become your portfolio; the others can be used for organising and storing notes for each unit, and for a 'college and course administration' file (see Figure 1.4, Filing your material)
- a **hole punch**
- **file paper**, plain and lined

▶ **plastic pockets** or **report files**. These are not essential but you may feel better if finished assignments are presented neatly in a binder or pocket of some sort. However, do not enclose each individual sheet of an assignment within a plastic pocket. This is expensive, ecologically unsound and drives your teachers and assessors crazy when they have to remove sheets to make comments on your work!

▶ **post-it index stickers** can be useful to help flag up important pieces of work, such as evidence for Key Skills certification

▶ **small exercise books** or **notebooks**, to act as logbooks or diaries

▶ a supply of **floppy disks** if you anticipate using a computer to word-process assignments and/or notes.

**Figure 1.4** *Filing your material*

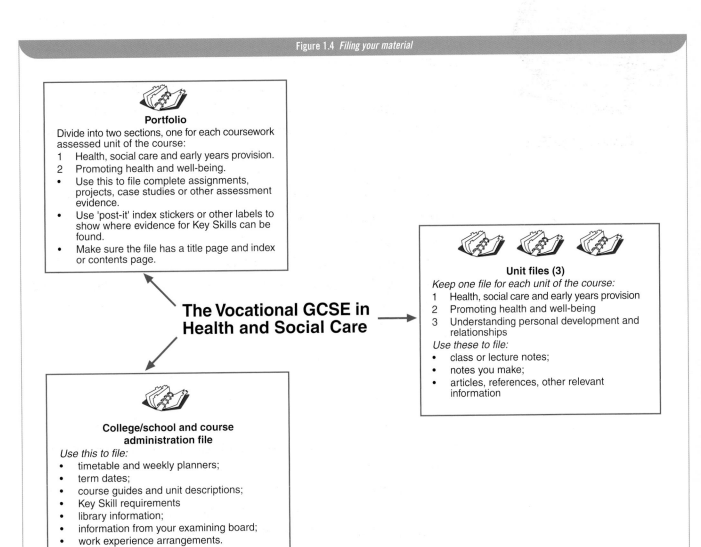

**Portfolio**
Divide into two sections, one for each coursework assessed unit of the course:
1   Health, social care and early years provision.
2   Promoting health and well-being.
• Use this to file complete assignments, projects, case studies or other assessment evidence.
• Use 'post-it' index stickers or other labels to show where evidence for Key Skills can be found.
• Make sure the file has a title page and index or contents page.

**Unit files (3)**
*Keep one file for each unit of the course:*
1   Health, social care and early years provision
2   Promoting health and well-being
3   Understanding personal development and relationships
*Use these to file:*
• class or lecture notes;
• notes you make;
• articles, references, other relevant information

**The Vocational GCSE in Health and Social Care**

**College/school and course administration file**
*Use this to file:*
• timetable and weekly planners;
• term dates;
• course guides and unit descriptions;
• Key Skill requirements
• library information;
• information from your examining board;
• work experience arrangements.

If you are dyslexic or have a disability which prevents or makes it difficult for you to take notes in lectures, you might consider acquiring a **small tape recorder** and a supply of **audio tapes** to enable you to record lectures and play them back at another time.

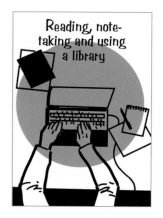

# READING, NOTE-TAKING AND USING A LIBRARY

Textbooks such as this can offer you a basic framework for the ideas and information you need for the different subject areas covered in the Vocational GCSE in Health and Social Care.

Your lectures and classes will supply you with additional material. However, you will need to carry out your own **reading and research**, making your own notes and updating information in areas where there is constant change (such as social policy legislation, or health advice). It will be useful for you to find out how the national organisation of health and care services works in the area and communities in which you live.

You cannot do this successfully without making full use of **libraries** (including their computers), **newspapers** and **journals**, **television** and **film**, and information produced by a range of national, local and voluntary organisations. If your have personal access to the **Internet**, you may find such research decidedly easier. Make sure that you are shown how to use all the relevant facilities of your library/learning centre, whether school, college or public. Use the checklist on page 13 to ensure that you are aware of all the resources on offer.

## Using the Internet

Think before reaching for the mouse. Using the Internet can be highly productive but it can take up a lot of your time. Before you start, work out:

▶ what you need to know

▶ how much you need to know

▶ when you need the information by

▶ whether you have a sensible search strategy. Do you have a list of recommended sites or know how to use an appropriate **search engine**, such as Yahoo, Lycos or Google? Try to narrow down the area that you are studying. For example, typing in 'HIV' on a search engine will bring up literally thousands of sites to choose from. Be more specific. For example, if you are preparing a poster for students about HIV, try typing in 'Health advice teenagers HIV UK.' A useful tip is to type in KS4 (Key Stage 4) after whatever topic you are investigating. This will bring up sites that contain material accessible to GSCE students.

▶ Could you find the information you need more easily in books or a journal?

Between them, the five sites listed below contain links to literally hundreds of the main health and social care organisations in this country. They are an excellent place from which to start any research.

▶ National Institute for Social Work at www.nisw.org.uk/

▶ Office for National Statistics at www.ons.gov.uk/

▶ King's Fund at www.kingsfund.org.uk/

▶ Government Information Service at www.open.gov.uk

▶ National Health Service at www.doh.gov.uk

---

**IN MY LIBRARY I CAN:**

● find all shelving where there are books and journals relevant to the subjects covered in this course ☐

*Make a note of the shelving reference numbers (usually the Dewey System) for health and social care books, sociology, psychology and biology books.*

● use the library's cataloguing and reference facilities, both manual and computerised. ☐

● operate the photocopying facilities. ☐

● order books and use any short-term loan arrangement. ☐

● find and use appropriate reference books, such as the British Humanities Index or Social Trends, to look up research, articles and statistics relevant to my assignments. ☐

● access the Internet and download useful material. ☐

● use CD-ROM facilities for research, e.g. to search through the broadsheet newspapers on disk for relevant articles/information. ☐

● use the reference section to look up names/addresses and phone numbers of local and national health and social care organisations ☐

● find my library membership card! ☐

Table 1.3 *Checklist for using a library*

# Strategies for reading

It is helpful to think of four types of reading: **receptive** and **reflective reading**, **skimming** and **scanning**. All types are useful at some stage in your reading.

1. **Receptive reading** is the reading you do most commonly. You use this method when reading for pleasure. Reading takes place at a steady pace and what is being read is fairly easy to absorb and understand. You may be able to use this type of reading for novels and magazine articles generally related to some of the themes and issues covered in the course.

2. **Reflective reading** is reading for information. This occurs when you have to think a little more carefully about what you are reading, perhaps because the vocabulary, ideas or information contained in it are new or difficult. There may be a lot of information presented. You may need to evaluate what you are reading and this may cause you to pause frequently to think about the material.

3. **Skimming** through a text, running your eyes down the page fairly rapidly, can give you a good impression of what the material is about. This is a useful technique when you need to consider whether or not to spend time reading the material more closely.

4. **Scanning** also involves running your eyes over a text, but in this case you are looking for particular points. Use this when looking for answers to particular questions or for specific references.

   To be of most use to you, reading will often need to be combined with **note-taking**.

# Note-taking strategies

Taking notes is time-consuming and requires active concentration. Students often worry when:

▸ they are spending too much time taking endless detailed notes without really understanding what they will use the notes for

▸ they give up note-taking because they cannot seem to work out what to write down and what to leave out. This can be a particular problem when taking notes in lessons and lectures.

## Why take notes?

Essentially, note-taking is a strategy for helping you **think**, **understand** and **remember**. There are many situations in life when it is important to focus on the **key issues** or points being communicated. A nurse may have to listen carefully to a patient describing the symptoms of an illness, and later relay this information to other medical staff. A nursery nurse may have to know exactly what to do if a child in her care has an asthma attack or needs adrenaline for a peanut allergy. She may have to explain these things quickly to another person, **summarising** essential information. Both of these health and care workers will have used mental and/or written note-taking skills, the nurse as she is listening to the patient, and the nursery nurse when she initially studied the first-aid procedures to apply in emergencies.

Deciding what to write down when you take notes is easier if you think about why you are taking notes. You may need to take different types of notes for different reasons. You will get better at working out methods of note-taking which suit you the more you try

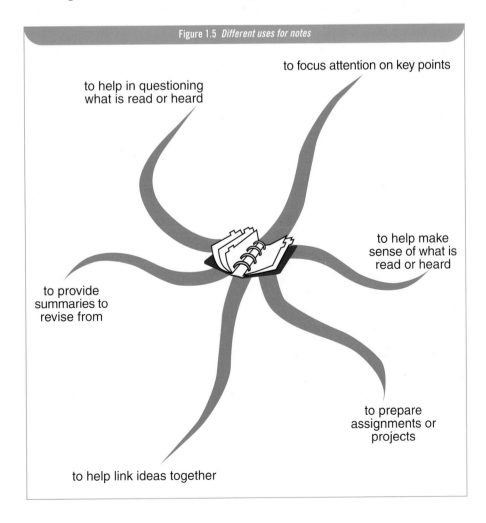

Figure 1.5 *Different uses for notes*

to focus attention on key points

to help in questioning what is read or heard

to help make sense of what is read or heard

to provide summaries to revise from

to prepare assignments or projects

to help link ideas together

out different approaches. It also helps to think about ways to store your notes so that they are easily accessible to you when you need them. If they are written or designed in such a way that you can make use of them again, you are more likely to come back to them.

Three useful methods for taking notes are:

▶ mind-mapping

▶ underlining and highlighting

▶ PQ4R.

*Mind-mapping*

Visual thinkers may find this technique extremely useful for summarising key points and issues.

▶ In the centre of your page, draw a picture or write your main topic or theme.

▶ Draw branches from this main topic in thick lines (use different colours or patterns). Label your branches with key words and/or images.

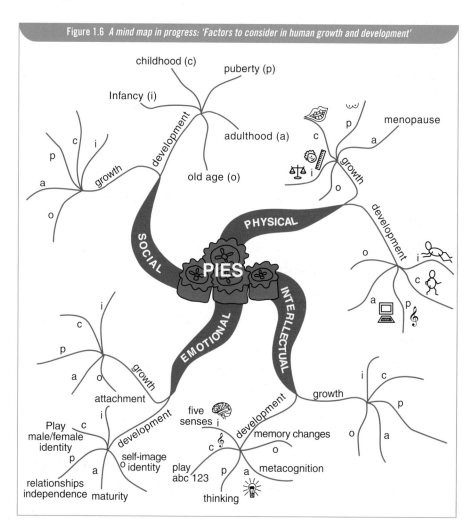

**Figure 1.6** *A mind map in progress: 'Factors to consider in human growth and development'*

❱ Draw sub-branches from the main branches to represent sub-topics or to elaborate and extend your ideas. Again, use key words, phrases, images, symbols, pictures and colour. Use *italics*, <u>underlining</u> and CAPITALS to highlight your work.

Let your ideas flow and develop. Add more details to your mind map as ideas or questions occur to you. However, the mind map is not meant to be an art form, more a way to focus your attention on the essential components of a piece of work, topic or report.

### Underlining and highlighting

If you own the book or article you are taking notes from, highlighting, underlining and marking the margin with asterisks or other symbols can be a quick and effective method of skim-reading a text, focusing your attention on it and getting to grips with the material as a whole.

### PQ4R

Linear and sequential thinkers (those who like to plot the logical connections between items of information or arguments) may find the note-taking method known as PQ4R worth using.

P  Preview

Q  Question

R  Read

R  Reflect

R  Recite

R  Review

❱ **Preview** – Before you begin to read your chapter, article, web page or book:

  ▸ Stop! Look at the title, author name, contents page and the date the text was published.

  ▸ Read any introduction.

  ▸ Scan the section you are reading for headings, subheadings and key passages.

  ▸ Look at the pictures, charts, graphs and other visual images.

❱ **Question** – Now ask yourself:

  ▸ What do I already know about this topic/issue/idea?

  ▸ What do I need to know?

  ▸ What am I likely to learn from this text? What **questions** is the author addressing? What information is given?

▸ Will I need to extract a little or a lot of information from this material? How useful will the information be to me?

▸ Where in this text will I find what I need to know? Do I have to read/take notes from all of it?

▸ **Read** – Read carefully through the material, **rereading** difficult passages. Stop and think about what you have read.

▸ **Reflect** – Make notes on the **key information** or ideas in the text. As you do so, question what you note down. Do you agree with what you are reading? Do you think the author has missed important points, evidence or issues? Which points/information seem particularly important or crucial? Are there terms, names, or dates that you think you may need to remember or come back to? Are there any ideas or information that would help you to write an assignment? Has something the author has written helped you to understand another issue?

▸ **Recite** – If the text you are making notes on contains information you need to memorise, without looking at the text, **recite** quietly the main points to yourself. Reread the text or your notes if you cannot do this.

▸ **Review** – Check, when trying to recall the main points of a text, that your notes make sense. You may need to make a **shorter summary** of your longer notes. Use coloured pens and symbols; jot down key words and phrases, diagrams or sketches on to a small card (card or index files can help). Now try to convert these shortened notes into your own words, either orally or in writing.

# Activity

Working individually or as small group, experiment with the three different methods for taking notes described above.

▸ Take notes from a page or two of this textbook.
▸ Take notes from a lecture or lesson.
▸ Take notes from a relevant television documentary.

Discuss and compare the results of your experiments using each method. Which method did you feel most comfortable with? Did you find yourself writing too little or too much? How much time did the exercise take? Would you find the notes useful to read again? What would you use the notes for?

It is sometimes said that we now live in a world of **information overload**. The growth of the mass media and, in particular, the Internet, means we are bombarded daily with information, ideas and viewpoints from a huge number of sources. The ability to extract what is useful and discard what is not from what you read, see and hear is essential to avoid overload and confusion. Note-taking can help you acquire this skill.

# WRITING ASSIGNMENTS, PROJECTS AND CASE STUDIES

## Why assess through coursework?

Two-thirds of the Vocational GCSE in Health and Social Care is assessed through coursework. Most of the coursework is set in the form of assignments, projects or case studies. Why is your work being assessed in this way, rather than, for instance, through examinations? There are four main reasons.

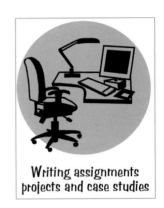

Writing assignments projects and case studies

1. To allow you to **make your own contribution to** each subject or topic-related assignment.

2. To help you acquire a **deeper knowledge and understanding** of the area you are studying.

3. To provide opportunities to **work with others** and **gain confidence** in approaching your teachers, tutors, friends and others working in health and social care organisations for help, extra information, work experience and the acquisition of practical skills.

4. To encourage you to use your own initiative in solving problems, answering questions and completing tasks set. Ultimately, to put you **in charge of your own learning**. To enable you to work out, after you have finished a piece of work, what you have learnt and what you still need to know, what was easy and what was more difficult and how you would improve it given another chance. To enable you to know when your work is good or good enough without over-relying on the approval and assessments of others. Finally, to allow you to transfer appropriate skills and knowledge to any future study or work. When you can do this you will have well-developed **meta-cognitive skills**, i.e. you can 'think about thinking' and reflect critically on the ways you learn, choosing strategies most appropriate to a task.

# Starting an assignment

Working out what an assignment requires you to do needs to be approached actively and positively.

Ask yourself these questions:

▶ Why am I doing this?

▶ What do I have to do here?

▶ What will be the best way to approach this task?

▶ What kind(s) of writing will the task involve? Will I be asked to:

  ▸ give an account of something?

  ▸ explain something?

  ▸ provide information about an issue?

  ▸ persuade?

  ▸ discuss different views?

  ▸ analyse and evaluate?

▶ Do I need to change the way I am tackling this piece of work?

▶ How can I improve what I am doing?

▶ Have I other skills I could use to help with this task?

Because they use **technical** or **specialist vocabulary**, assignments can sometimes be written in ways that make it difficult to work out what to do and how to begin.

Look at these three typical assignment tasks:

1. **Analyse** the different ways in which people cope with life-changes. What types of help and support might people need to manage these life-changes?

2. **Analyse** the effectiveness of codes of practice and charters in upholding the care value base.

3. **Evaluate** your communication strategies accurately, identifying strengths and ways to improve on weaknesses.

If you are unsure what is meant by words such as **analyse** and **evaluate**, use the *Key words and phrases table* on page 21 to help you work out what is required.

**Brainstorm** the wording of the task, trying to note down anything you think might be relevant.

For example, '**Analyse** the effectiveness of codes of practice and charters in upholding the care value base.'

The result of a brainstorm exercise on this task might look like Figure 1.7.

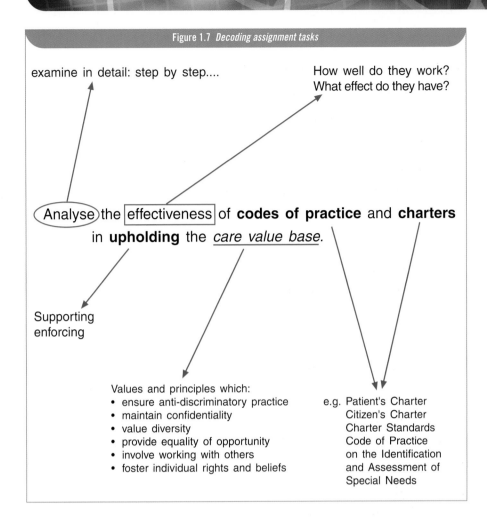

Figure 1.7 *Decoding assignment tasks*

examine in detail: step by step....

How well do they work?
What effect do they have?

(Analyse) the [effectiveness] of **codes of practice** and **charters** in **upholding** the *care value base*.

Supporting
enforcing

Values and principles which:
• ensure anti-discriminatory practice
• maintain confidentiality
• value diversity
• provide equality of opportunity
• involve working with others
• foster individual rights and beliefs

e.g. Patient's Charter
Citizen's Charter
Charter Standards
Code of Practice
on the Identification
and Assessment of
Special Needs

Table 1.4 *Key words and phrases*

● **Analyse**    examine in detail; separate into component parts
*If we analyse our survey of teenage smoking, we find that girls generally start smoking at an earlier age than boys.*

● **Compare**    looks for differences and similarities
*A comparison of the Sex Discrimination and Race Relations Act shows that they both make a distinction between indirect and direct discrimination.*

● **Critically evaluate**    use evidence to support your judgements
*Mary's critical evaluation of child poverty in Britain discussed evidence from large- and small-scale research studies.*

● **Describe**    give a written, visual or oral account, as required
*I described the Greentrees Home for the Elderly as well-resourced, warm and welcoming, sympathetic to the needs of its occupants and forward thinking.*

● **Explain**    make clear and give reasons for; help others understand
*Most teenagers would benefit from an exact explanation of the effects of oestrogen and progesterone on the body during puberty.*

● **Identify**    pick out key characteristics: What is most important?
*Ishmael identified the key characteristics of a good piece of research as readability, validity and relevance.*

● **Discuss**    consider an issue from various points of view
*In my report I discussed different views on the use of "politically correct" language in health and care work.*

## Activity

Now carry out a similar decoding exercise for the other assignment tasks (or others you have been given by your school/college). If you are working in a group or class, compare and discuss your interpretation of the questions.

# Organising ideas and action planning

When you have worked out what the assignment requires you to do, you need to consider:

◗ how to collect the information you need. Where will you find suitable information or source material? Who can help you or give you the information you need? What range of sources will you be expected to use?

◗ how, if you are working as a group, you will hold meetings and share out the tasks.

Brainstorming, spider diagrams and mind-mapping are three techniques for organising and generating ideas.

1. **Brainstorming** is particularly useful if you are working in a group. Simply note down any useful ideas, words, visual images, arguments or information relevant to the question being discussed.

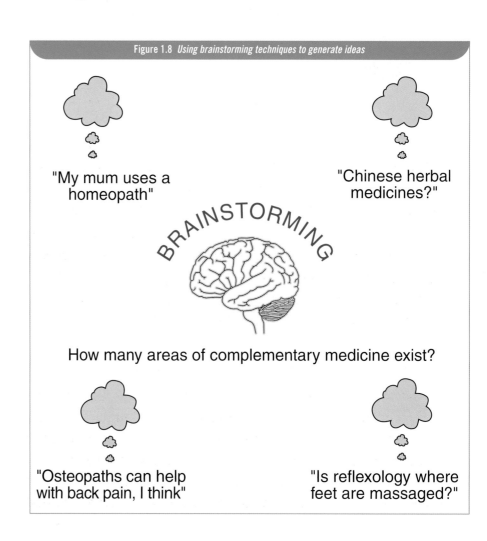

Figure 1.8 *Using brainstorming techniques to generate ideas*

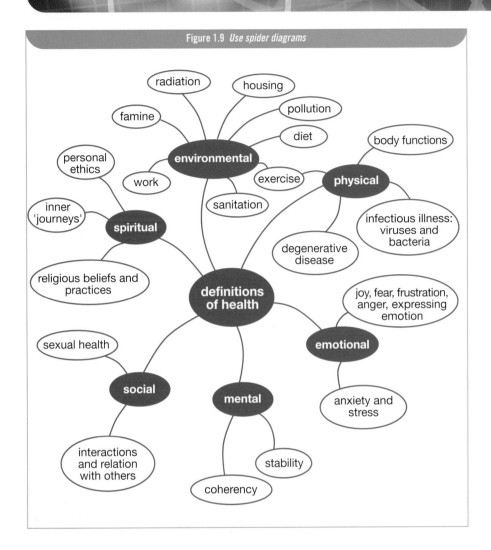

**Figure 1.9** *Use spider diagrams*

2. **Spider diagrams** are helpful if you haven't much time and need a rough sketch of what a piece of work might involve. They can help you begin to structure and link material and ideas together.

3. **Mind-mapping**, described in more detail on page 16, is a very useful technique for visual learners who find it easier to organise their thoughts and ideas in linked key words and pictures. This method can be used for generating ideas and planning your work as well as, later on, note-taking and revising.

## Planning and prioritising tasks

If you use a planner regularly it is easier to break up assignments and projects into a series of smaller tasks, each of which you could aim to complete within a manageable time, such as an hour or two. Subdividing your work in this way also allows you to prioritise the tasks. In what order are they best done? Which really need to be done straightaway? Make a list of small tasks in order of prior-

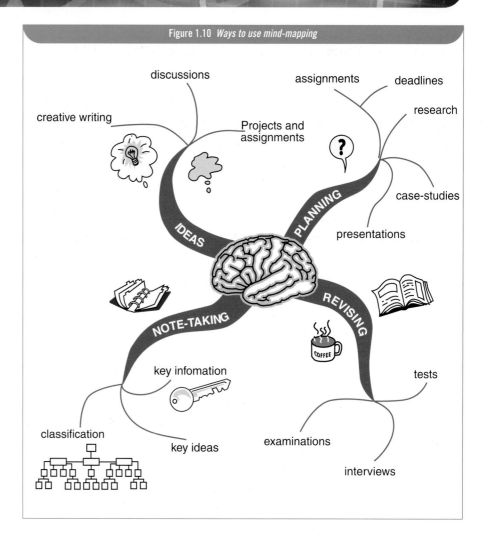

**Figure 1.10** *Ways to use mind-mapping*

ity, noting the time you estimate they will take and target dates for completion. Leave room on your action plan to amend these dates when and if your plan is modified.

## Example: Breaking down an assignment into smaller tasks

Nadia has been asked to complete the following assignment. She has been given almost a term (ten weeks) to complete the assignment.

Present a profile of two different health and/or social care and/or early years services. You must include:

▶ how each service is organised and funded

▶ the roles of the people who work in each service

▶ how the care value base is applied by care workers

▶ ways in which each service meets the care needs of individuals

▶ barriers that could prevent clients from using the services.

(This was adapted from OCR specifications for the Health, Social Care and Early Years Provision, Double Award GCSE. 2002)

## Nadia's action plan

▶ Decide which two services to choose for the assignment. Arrange to discuss this with tutor at college. Will probably choose to look at **day nurseries** for one of the services because I'm arranging to spend a week at a nursery next month.

*Time 20 minutes*                    Complete by: 2 October

▶ Have decided to study **day nurseries** and the **local community project for older people**. Write to the community project to arrange a visit there before the end of November. Confirm work experience arrangements at the nursery.

*Time: 1 hour*                    Complete by: 15 October

▶ Make notes on the **care value base** from my textbook and class notes.

*Time: 1 hour*                    Complete by: 22 October

▶ Prepare my **interview schedules** for the visit to the community project and the nursery. Use my class notes and textbook for ideas about the questions to include. Type up interview schedules. Ask tutor to check them for me. Read the notes I took from my textbook about **preparing for a work experience placement** [see pages 46–47 of this book] and make sure I have completed all preparation tasks.

*Time: 3 hours*                    Complete by: 29 October

▶ Make sure I have **film in my camera** so I can take photos of people at the nursery and at the community centre.

*Time: 10 minutes*                    Complete by: 5 November

▶ **Spend week at nursery**. Keep **logbook**. Make sure I find as much information as possible about organisation, funding, staffing and how the care value base is applied.

*Time: 1 week: 12–16 November*

Complete all my notes by 22 November

▶ **Spend day at community centre** for older people. Carry out interview with manager, talk to users of the service and find out as much as I can about the organisation.

Write up notes.

*Time: 1 day: 25th November*

Complete all my notes by 28 November

▶ Ask tutor for help in how to find more general information about the **local and national organisation of day nurseries and community projects** for older people. Make notes for my assignment.

*Time: 4 hours*                    Complete by 12 December

▶ **Write first draft of whole assignment** using my computer. Use proofreading techniques and computer spell-checker to correct errors.

*Time: 4–5 hours*                    Complete by 18 December

▶ Show first draft to my tutor. Ask for her comments. Make changes. **Hand in final draft of completed assignment.**

*Time: 40 minutes*
Complete by 20 December

*Total time I need*: Approx. *6 days work experience/visits* plus another *16 hours* for study and writing/typing up work.

## Monitoring and revising your work

There are likely to be many points during the completion of a piece of coursework when you will change direction or modify your original plan in some way. On your action plan, keep a note of:

▶ the reasons for changing your plans
▶ what new plans you have for the work.

## Writing skills

When you have reached the point when you want to start writing the assignment, you need to think about the quality of the language that you will use to convey your ideas. Problems can crop up when:

▶ you are unsure whether the assignment should be written in an academic, formal style ('it can be argued that…'), or whether it is acceptable to use the first person ('I found that…'). Check with the person who set the assignment.

▶ you have difficulty with the **flow** of the writing, especially when evaluating or analysing an issue from several different perspectives or when there is a lot of conflicting evidence. Use the *linking words and phrases* checklist in Table 1.5 below to help you write an introduction and link each paragraph to the next one, introducing new ideas and points in a clear way without losing sight of the original aims of the report.

# Activity

Use the example of Nadia's action plan to help you prepare an action plan for your first set assignment. You may find that your school or college will give you an action-planning form to fill in for each assignment. If not, it will be quite acceptable for you to invent your own along the lines of the example above. Use your IT skills to prepare a format which you could use to save time on each new piece of work.

▶ you reach the end of the report and need to draw ideas together and write a conclusion and/or evaluation. You need to avoid abrupt, over-brief evaluations. Use *A guide to VGCSE evaluation* below to show that you have reflected upon and analysed the issues involved, as well as considered your own performance.

## A guide to Vocational GCSE evaluation

**Evaluating** a piece of work is not necessarily the same as **concluding** it. When writing a **conclusion** to an assignment, the key issues or experiences discussed in the work can be fully summarised and, depending on the kind of assignment or project, judgement may be made about the validity or reliability of the theories or evidence discussed. The ideas and knowledge covered by the

---

**INTRODUCTORY PARAGRAPHS**

In this report/assignment/case study I intend to...
This report will discuss/analyse/examine/compare/evaluate...
There are two/three/four theories which need to be considered...
There are several areas of this debate...

**CONNECTING EACH POINT AND/OR PARAGRAPH**

It can be argued that...
Some writers suggest that...
Nevertheless...
On the other hand...
At first sight...
"X" argues that..., whereas "y" suggests that...
Caution needs to be exercised in interpreting these results because...
In his/her discussion/analysis of...
Arguably...
What is interesting about this view is...
The theory implies that...
As we have seen...

**CONCLUDING REMARKS**

In conclusion...
This evidence/research confirms that...
There is insufficient evidence in the research to...
While this policy has benefited..., it has been of less value to ...

To summarise...
In short...
What this idea fails to recognise is...

*Table 1.5  Checklist of linking words and phrases*

course can be complex. Good conclusions should reflect the fact that different points of view exist and different solutions to problems need to be assessed.

**Evaluating** a piece of work offers you the opportunity to take another look at **how** you completed the assignment. You may be asked to consider whether the way in which you tackled the work was appropriate. Can you justify the approach you took to the work? Could you have done the work differently? What could you have done to improve the work?

You are being encouraged to look critically at your own learning and performance on the course. It is important to realise that you are not expected to produce perfect work from the very beginning of your studies. However, if you take the time to evaluate your work carefully, you will soon become much more aware of the ways in which your knowledge, skills and understanding can improve.

When evaluating a coursework assignment you should consider the following:

▶ Check the original requirements of the assignment. Have you met them all? Show the ways in which you could have done so.

▶ What approaches to the assignment did you consider and which did you actually use? Which worked well and which did not? Why?

▶ What skills does your assignment demonstrate?

▶ What improvements would you make if you did this piece of work again and why?

## Proofreading your work

At this level of study it is not acceptable to hand in first drafts of work. Presentation is important (just as it would be if you were preparing a report in the workplace). You will be expected to check your own work for errors. The use of a dictionary, spellchecker and thesaurus should become automatic. Students with spelling or word-finding difficulties could consider the use of a hand-held electronic spellchecker. These are relatively inexpensive (£12.00–£30.00) and some models also include a thesaurus (i.e. a list of words with similar meanings), a calculator, games, grammar guides, etc.) Franklin makes some of the best models, which are easily available from high-street stores such as Argos. If you are dyslexic and standard spellchecking programmes do not pick up all your errors, there are some useful software applications. See the resources section on pages 51–52 for more details.

### How to proofread

Proofreading is the process of rereading your work, looking for and correcting mistakes. You can look for different types of mistakes, such as:

▶ missing capital letters

▶ capitals where there shouldn't be capitals

▶ missing full stops, commas or other kinds of punctuation

▶ sentences that don't make sense

▶ spelling mistakes.

**Proofreading** can be easier if you:

▶ leave some time between doing the writing and proofreading it – this makes it easier to spot the mistakes

▶ proofread for one kind of a mistake at a time – you may miss a lot if you try to correct everything at once

▶ try starting with the last word, then check the second-to-last word, and so on, when proofreading for spelling mistakes. This makes spelling mistakes jump out at you much more

▶ decide how much proofreading you really need to do. Some pieces of work, like assignments, projects and case studies, do need very careful proofreading. Other work, like a note you have written for yourself, just needs checking to ensure that it makes sense.

## Presentation skills

How much care do you take over the presentation of your work? Use Table 1.6 to work out your own strengths and weaknesses. On this course, you will also be actively encouraged to develop skills in the use of information technology. Typing or word processing all or part of your assignments is much easier if you can touch-type. See the resources section on pages 51–52 for information about good touch-typing programmes. However, practice in using the keyboard, using both hands, should enable you to type fast enough to make word-processing your work worthwhile.

When I look through my work I notice that:     (Tick any that apply to you)

1  I usually put the **date** of the work. ☐

2  I usually make sure my work has a **title** and it is **underlined**. ☐

3  My writing is **legible** or I **type** my work. Other people can easily read what I have written. ☐

4  I **do not** leave **large gaps or spaces** between sections of my writing. ☐

5  If I need to number my work, the **numbering is clear**. ☐

6  I draw **clear diagrams** and **tables**. ☐

7  I always **label** my diagrams and tables neatly, using a ruler where necessary. ☐

8  I use plenty of **colour** in my pictures and illustrations. ☐

9  **Loose worksheets** are **attached carefully** to my books or files. ☐

10  **I finish off any work at home** which I did not have time to finish in class. ☐

11  I try to **correct my own work**, proofreading or redrafting pieces of work before I hand them in to be marked. ☐

12  **I correct my own spelling mistakes**, using a spellchecker, or asking someone to help me. ☐

13  **Good presentation of my work** seems to help me achieve better grades. ☐

*Table 1.6  Presentation skills*

# Writing a bibliography

You will need to write a bibliography (a list of books, articles and other resources used) for each assignment you submit. To do this properly, you need to make a note of your materials and references as you study. There is nothing worse than finishing an assignment and then spending valuable time hunting down the name of a book you read in the library but did not note down the details of. As a general rule, you need to note:

▶ the title of the book or article (or website address)

▶ the author(s)

▶ the publisher

▶ the date of publication

▶ the place of publication.

## Examples

*Book*

Thomson, H. and Aslangul, S. (2002) *Vocational GCSE Health and Social Care*, London, Hodder and Stoughton.

*Article*

Patmore, C. (2002), 'Help in Adversity', *Community Care Magazine*, 13 December–9 January 2002.

*An article or chapter from a 'reader'*

(i.e. a book containing many articles or chapters by different authors)

Tester, S (1996) 'Women and community care', *Women and Social Policy*. Ed. Hallett, C. London, Prentice Hall.

Other sources of information or references in your work may come from the Internet (give the **website** address), workplace (acknowledge the **source**), television programmes, video or film (give the **title and date**) or friends, family and teachers (**attribute** information as accurately as you can.)

# MEMORY SKILLS AND TECHNIQUES

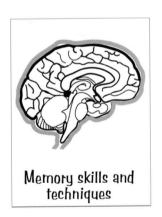

**Memory skills and techniques**

One unit of the Vocational GCSE in Health and Social Care is externally assessed through a timed test. The Key Skills Qualification also involves external assessments, including some tests. There may also be occasions during your course when your teachers feel it is important to ask you to memorise material.

However, students taking this course will not be expected to write essays or lengthy, extended answers to questions under test conditions.

# Why have timed tests?

There are many situations like the one below in working life where, under pressure, it will be important or even crucial (for example, in giving first aid) to have memorised key information or ideas. In more routine working situations it will, of course, be possible, if necessary, to check one's understanding or memory by consulting reference manuals, books or colleagues. Skills become more automatic with practice. Nevertheless, being required to memorise something is good rehearsal for real-life pressures and crises. VGCSE tests are therefore designed to give you practice in:

▶ reviewing key information, ideas and theories

▶ developing and understanding effective memory techniques

▶ writing short responses to stimulus questions under timed test conditions.

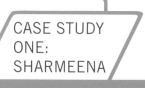

CASE STUDY ONE: SHARMEENA

Consider the following situation:

Sharmeena is a nursery nurse at a day nursery for under fives. Parents normally pick up the children at 5.30pm. On Friday, Paul, Josie's father, turns up fifteen minutes early, clearly drunk and demanding to take his daughter home immediately. Paul does not live with Josie's mother and there is an agreement that he picks up Josie on Mondays and Tuesdays, and Pat, Josie's mother, picks her up on the other three weekdays.

Sharmeena has answered the door to Paul, who is now shouting at her in the reception area of the nursery building. He is swearing and threatening to push Sharmeena out of the way if she does not let him into the room where the children are playing.

Though feeling nervous, Sharmeena has fortunately **remembered three key pieces of advice** given to her at a training course on facing aggression in the workplace:

● stay calm and use positive rather than negative words and phrases to help change the emotion of the aggressor

● offer to reward good behaviour

● firmly and gently explain how the aggressor's behaviour is affecting you.

Sharmeena suggests to Paul that she can help him if he stops shouting. She says that she will talk to her supervisor to see what she can do to help, adding that his shouting is making her feel nervous, although she is sure a solution to the problem can be found. Although still tense and red-faced, Paul calms down enough to listen to the nursery manager, who has now arrived at the scene. He agrees to wait to talk to Josie's mother and, in the intervening ten minutes, reveals that there have been problems between Pat and himself over access to Josie.

# Preparing for tests

## Overcoming examination nerves

We feel nervous when we do not feel confident. Tests and examinations put us under pressure to show what we can do or what we know. Our performance may be measured against the performance of other people around us. It would be strange, therefore, if we did not feel anxious!

Some anxiety is natural and may actually help us in tests and examinations. If we are keyed-up for a test, we are concentrating hard and focusing on what we have to do. We want to succeed. If we could not care less and are totally relaxed, we may not have enough adrenaline speeding through our system to keep us going throughout the test.

However, too much anxiety and nervousness can also be a problem. It can make our minds go blank just when we need to remember what we have learnt or when we need to concentrate on a problem. Some people feel most anxious about performance tests, such as a driving test or a piano examination. Other people worry more about written tests. A person may be good at remembering facts, but less confident about puzzling out which of several answers in a multiple-choice question is the best one to choose.

## Ensuring adequate preparation

One of the surest ways of avoiding too much panic is to allow enough time to **prepare carefully** for the tests.

▶ Make sure you know which of your course units will be externally tested and when the tests will take place. Will you be given another chance to take the tests if you do not do so well as you hoped the first time round?

▶ Gather all the information and advice you can find on what you need to learn for the test by consulting your course guide, your class notes, your textbooks, teachers and friends. Ask to see some practice test papers.

▶ Start the process of revision and review well in advance of the test date, using your weekly planner to assign short but regular 'chunks' of time to test preparation. Figure 1.11 *The importance of reviewing*, demonstrates how effective such regular boosts to your memory can be.

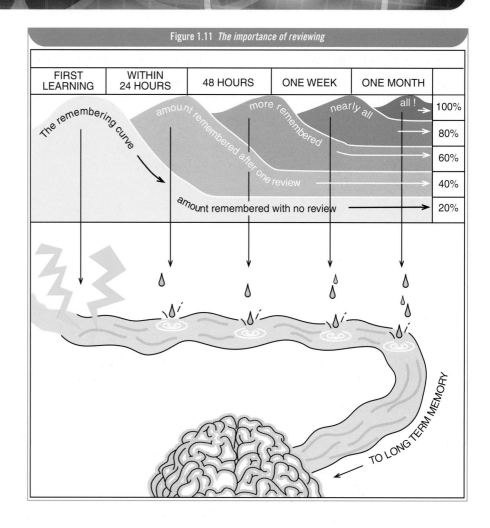

Figure 1.11 *The importance of reviewing*

## Activity

Try out the theory demonstrated in Figure 1.11 yourself. Over a period of a month, choose a particular section of information that you need to learn for a test. Plot out, on your weekly planner or diary, fifteen minutes for revision of this material within 24 hours, 28 hours, one week and a month of first trying to learn it. Try to keep to this revision plan and, at the end, assess whether the material has been learned effectively.

(Alternatively, persuade a teacher or lecturer to build this experimental exercise into their class time).

## Understanding memory

Explore different methods for remembering your material (see Figure 1.12 *Make your memory work!*). Information can be remembered in many ways and finding strategies which work for you will give you an insight into how your memory works and how you can use it more effectively. Refer back to the section of this chapter on **learning styles** (page 3). Which methods of memorising information might best suit your preferred learning styles?

# Activity

Look at Table 1.7 *Legislation and organisations which challenge discrimination* for five minutes. Try to remember as much as you can without writing anything down. Now cover the table and try to write down everything you remember.

In groups or individually, discuss and consider the following:

▶ Which strategies did you use to remember the contents of the table? Did they include any of the strategies described in Figure 1.12?
▶ What additional strategies (written, verbal, other) might have been effective?
▶ What would you need to do to retain this information for a test in a month's time?

| Table 1.7 *Legislation and organisations which challenge discrimination* | | |
|---|---|---|
| Sex Discrimination Act 1975 | The Commission for Racial Equality | Disability Discrimination Act 1995 |
| The European Court of Justice | The Equal Opportunities Commission | The European Convention of Human Rights |
| Race Relations Act 1976 | The Disability Rights Commission | Fair Employment Act (Northern Ireland) 1989 |

Figure 1.12 *Make your memory work!*

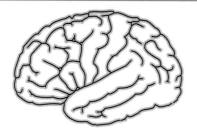

# Make Your Memory Work!

### Speech
Talk through and explain to someone else what you have learnt. Put the material on tape and listen to it. Write questions for yourself and ask someone to test you.

### Association
Use **grouping** and **chunking** techniques to associate sets of information or ideas.

### Imagination
The *Cicero's Rooms* technique can be used for remembering up to ten pieces of information or key facts.
This is a visualising technique which involes imagining yourself moving from room to room in your home, 'placing' each fact or piece of information somewhere in a room as you go. When you try to recall the facts, go back through the rooms in your mind, 'seeing' the information you left there.

### Movement
Walk around or play relaxing music. Pace up and down while trying to learn something.

## Use mind-mapping

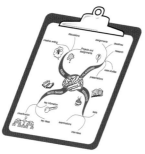

### Mnemonics
Use visual and auditory mnemonics.

**Visual**

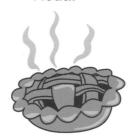

**Auditory**

4  key aspects of growth and development.
P  physical
I  intellectual
E  emotional
S  social

### Order
Use linking strategies. Work out ways in which ideas or information can be linked together, or one paragraph of key material associated with the next. For information involving dates, timelines can help. Some people enjoy inventing short stories to help them remember key facts.

### Repetition
Rewrite and condense material several times until the key points are remembered. Review and re-test yourself at regular intervals. Work for a maximum of 20 minutes at a time. Take a break. Start again.

### Symbolism
Condense information into its bare essentials. Use acronyms (e.g. C.R.E. for Commission for Racial Equality) and dates.
Put this super-condensed information on small cards and use for last-minute revision before the exam.

# Test techniques

▶ On the day of a test, arrive on time but not too early, giving yourself plenty of time to check equipment and to have something to eat beforehand.

▶ Try not to talk about the test with friends before you start.

▶ Have a last look at any brief notes or summaries you have made.

▶ As soon as you are allowed to, read the questions.

▶ Make sure you understand the test instructions. Ask for help if necessary.

▶ Take your time.

▶ Highlight key words and note down any key facts you know you will have to use at some point but may forget as the test proceeds.

▶ If you suffer from acute 'nerves', give yourself something to smile about and imagine (just briefly!) the teachers in charge of the examination in a nudist camp. If all else fails, take a few deep breaths and tell yourself you are not going to let the test get the better of you. Start with the questions you feel most confident with and then tackle the rest.

▶ Answer all the questions.

▶ Time and pace yourself. Keep an eye on the clock or a watch. Be strict about keeping within time limits for the questions.

▶ Leave time at the end of the test to proofread and check your answers.

Keep tests in perspective. It will be great if you do well because you will enjoy feeling successful, but if you do not, it is not the end of the world. You can always do things differently next time.

# Special assessment concessions

The teachers of students with certain disabilities, illnesses or exceptional circumstances (including dyslexic and dyspraxic students) can, on their behalf, make a request to the examining board for special test arrangements (such as extra time) and/or special consideration (action taken after the examination). If you think you are eligible for, and could benefit from these concessions, discuss this with your teachers or tutors as far in advance of the tests as possible, preferably at the beginning of your course.

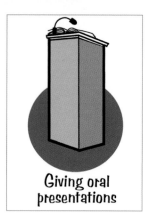

**Giving oral presentations**

# GIVING ORAL PRESENTATIONS

## CASE STUDY TWO: LENA

Lena has coped well with assignments, tests and work experience. Then she is asked to give a short oral presentation to her class on the research project she has been carrying out. Her friend Adam said that when he did his talk he quite enjoyed the chance to speak uninterrupted for a full ten minutes. Lena, however, would rather be forced to commit the entire NHS and Community Care Act to memory than stand up and speak in front of an audience, even one she knows as well as her GCSE group.

## Activity

1. Are you a Lena or an Adam (or perhaps something in between)? What advice would you offer to Lena so that she can overcome her nervousness and to Adam so that he can avoid giving a rambling or boring talk?

2. You may well be given the opportunity to give a short talk or presentation to enable you to develop greater self-confidence and to acquire a skill often used in working in health and social care occupations. For example, a ward manager in a hospital may have to brief doctors and paramedics about the condition of patients in her care, and a social worker may have to talk to groups of prospective foster parents. Can you think of other situations where health and social care workers may need to address groups of colleagues, clients, patients, service-users or the general public?

## Preparing a presentation

▶ Think about the purpose of the presentation. In what ways should your audience benefit from the talk?

▶ Are you hoping to give them information, or do you hope to discuss ideas and theories? Do you want your audience to participate in your presentation, or is the purpose of the talk to give a briefing? How will you keep your listeners interested in what you say? Will you use handouts or audiovisual aids, such as music, tape recordings, video/TV clips or a PowerPoint presentation? If so, you will need to ensure that the equipment is ready and set up for you to use.

▶ Consider the length of the presentation and practice what you want to say in that time. Try not to overrun your allotted time.

▶ Try not to read out from a script. Instead, make notes of the key points you want to make on cue cards and practise using these to put together your talk. A punchy and interesting introduction and conclusion to the talk always helps.

▶ Make sure you research and prepare your material carefully and stick to the 'brief' you are given for the talk.

▶ If you feel very nervous about giving a presentation alone, ask if you could 'pair up' with a fellow student to give a joint talk.

## Delivery of the talk

▶ It can be very helpful to use **cueing words** throughout your talk to help it flow along. You will probably use some of these automatically, but a quick glance at Table 1.8, *Delivering a talk using cues and signals*, may help you to choose some other useful phrases.

▶ Consider your posture and movements as you talk. Will you need to stand or sit, stay in one place or move around the room?

▶ Try to speak clearly, and avoid fixing your gaze on one or two people, especially your friends! Try to make everyone in the room feel included in your presentation.

## Confidence and self-esteem

Even if, like Lena in the story above, you are nervous **before** the talk, after it is over you should feel a great sense of **achievement**. With luck you should not find it so difficult to contemplate doing another presentation. There are many techniques for handling nerves, including taking deep breaths before you start. Often, the first few words are the worst. Once you have begun speaking and are concentrating on your material, feelings of nervousness often recede or disappear and you find that you can complete the talk. There will be plenty of people in your group who feel exactly the same as you do about giving talks, and their sympathies will be with you!

Make sure that you are given the opportunity to discuss how the presentation went with a teacher or tutor. Your fellow students will also give you plenty of informal **feedback**, but it is sometimes helpful if they are encouraged to offer comments within the classroom.

**1 SEQUENCE SIGNALS** *(I'M PUTTING MY IDEAS IN AN ORDER.)*

| | |
|---|---|
| first, second, third | in the first place, second place etc. |
| then | next |
| before | now |
| after | while |
| until | last(ly) |
| during | since |
| always | later/earlier |

**2 ILLUSTRATION SIGNALS** *(THIS IS WHAT I MEAN)*

| | |
|---|---|
| for example | specifically |
| for instance | to illustrate |
| such as | much like |
| in the same way as | similar to |

**3 CONTINUATION SIGNALS** *(I'VE MORE IDEAS TO COME)*

| | | |
|---|---|---|
| and | also | another |
| again | furthermore | last of all |
| first of all | likewise | in addition |
| moreover | next | more |
| other | secondly | one reason |
| too | with | similarly |
| | | and finally |
| | | a final reason |

**4 CHANGE OF DIRECTION SIGNALS** *(WATCH OUT – I'M GOING BACK OVER SOMETHING)*

| | | |
|---|---|---|
| although | but | conversely |
| despite | different from | even though |
| however | in contrast | instead of |
| in spite of | nevertheless | otherwise |
| the opposite | on the contrary | on the other hand |
| rather | still | yet |
| while | though | |

**5 EMPHASIS SIGNALS** *(I'M SAYING SOMETHING IMPORTANT NOW)*

| | |
|---|---|
| a major development | it all boils down to |
| a significant factor | most of all |
| a key feature | more than anything else |
| remember that | it should be noted |
| above all | especially important |
| especially relevant | important to note |

*Table 1.8 Delivering a talk using cues and signals*

# WORKING COLLABORATIVELY

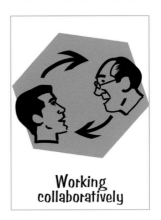

**Working collaboratively**

Television dramas such as *ER* and *Casualty* have provided us with vivid images of how positive, successful and sometimes essential it can be for health and care workers to work collaboratively, offering different skills and expertise and contributing ideas based on varied experiences and training. Most health and social care workers, whatever their individual roles and responsibilities, work as part of a wider team. Problems that affect staff and service users, patients or clients are discussed in meetings or supervision sessions. The improvement of the service as a whole becomes a shared responsibility.

However, it would not be true to claim that, within all health and care services, team or group work always operates effectively. Much depends on the **structure** of the organisation, the **size** of departments and the **hierarchies** within them, the type and quality of **management**, and **group dynamics**, i.e. how individuals within working groups or teams interact professionally and personally.

Some of these factors may affect the success of group-work assignments you may be asked to participate in. If your class or group has been encouraged, from the start of the course, to get to know each other well, to discuss issues in a non-threatening atmosphere of mutual respect and there have been many opportunities for whole- or small-group work, a group assignment is likely to be a productive and positive experience. It will also be an opportunity to develop and record evidence in the Key Skills of problem solving and working with others. Tables 1.9, 1.10 and 1.11 on pages 42–44 are designed to help you plan group-work projects, assessing your own skills and avoiding some of the pitfalls.

## Discussion

Well-managed class discussions can bring your course to life. Listening to and responding to other people's ideas can help you think through your own beliefs and opinions. Strong differences of opinion or perspective within a group can spark heated debate. A quieter, more thoughtful exchange of ideas can help you appreciate an issue or subject more clearly. Some people have few inhibitions about participating in discussions, but if just a few students dominate discussions they can become unsatisfactory and less enjoyable for the whole group.

Table 1.9 *How to work well in teams*

1 Allow problems in the group or team itself to be aired and discussed.

2 Make sure everyone in the team knows what the team has to do, has taken part in planning the work and understands their role.

3 Talk to each other!

4 Value everyone's contribution and role and encourage and praise each other's work.

5 If appropriate, give someone in the group a co-ordinating role.

6 Try not to allow groups or teams to become too big or too small.

7 Give yourself time to 'gel' as a group.

8 Make sure you have somewhere to work – a base – and, if necessary, somewhere to keep materials, equipment etc.

9 Discuss how you will make decisions and make them jointly. Be prepared to change or review your procedures.

10 Review regularly how the team is working and what progress it is making.

If you find it difficult to join in discussions, try the following strategies:

▶ **Listen** to a specific point the teacher or another student has made. **Ask a question, make a comment** about it or **offer an example or illustration** of it as early in the discussion as possible. When you have made a contribution, feelings of nervousness may recede and you may find it easier to contribute again.

▶ **Help others who are reluctant to contribute** by asking them questions, appealing to experiences or views you know they have. Try to share in the responsibility for keeping the discussion alive.

▶ Help the group to **stay focused on the subject** or purpose of the discussion, especially if there is a task to complete afterwards. If the discussion seems to be straying from the point, offer a contribution such as 'shall we go back to the question of…?', or 'So, there are two ways of looking at this…'

Discussions can also fall flat if only a few people in the group have bothered to read material suggested, or if participants allow personal problems between members of the group to affect the

The following statements reflect a wide range of possible roles. Which of these group roles do you generally take on?

| ROLE | MOST OF THE TIME | SOME OF THE TIME | NEVER |
|---|---|---|---|
| Acting as peacemaker, trying to smooth problems and reduce tension in the group | | | |
| Acting as the group clown or joker | | | |
| Being creative and original with ideas and views | | | |
| Being picked on or bullied by other group members | | | |
| Caring and looking after other group members who might be upset or uncomfortable | | | |
| Challenging and confronting views of behaviour of which you disapprove | | | |
| Constantly drawing others back to the task if they wander | | | |
| Constantly drawing the group back to its task or agenda | | | |
| Disrupting or sabotaging the formal agenda in order to follow your own | | | |
| Drawing out possible hidden agendas or feelings that may be blocking progress | | | |
| Encouraging and motivating others to contribute | | | |
| Encouraging others to be creative and original | | | |
| Initiating discussion or activities | | | |
| Keeping others focused on group task and purpose | | | |
| Listening quietly until you can see an opening to contribute | | | |
| Unhelpful stirring or winding other people up | | | |

**Table 1.10  Contributing to a group**

atmosphere and make it uncomfortable. Your teachers will probably be all too aware if this seems to be the case. It may be helpful to ask them to find ways to improve group dynamics.

| SUMMARY PERSONAL FEELINGS ABOUT GROUP PARTICIPATION | YOUR ASSESSMENT | OTHERS' ASSESSMENT, E.G. TEACHER/LECTURER/PEERS/ WORK-EXPERIENCE SUPERVISOR |
|---|---|---|
| Are you reasonably comfortable when taking part in a group activity or discussion? What reasons would you give for your answer? | | |
| What do you think that you contribute to a group, i.e. consider your strong points? | | |
| What difficulties or problems do you meet when in a group? | | |
| Are you confident of being able to lead or manage a group or group activity? | | |
| Have you the skills to lead or manage a group or group activity? | | |
| When contributing to, leading or managing a group do you always plan and prepare well? How important do you think it is to be well prepared? | | |
| What kind of leadership do you provide? | | |
| How effective is it? | | |
| How might you improve your leadership skills? | | |
| How do you think you could improve your contributions to a group and group-work skills? | | |

*Permission to reproduce this document is given by Stonham Housing Association Ltd*

Table 1.11 *Reviewing group-work skills*

# MANAGING WORK EXPERIENCE

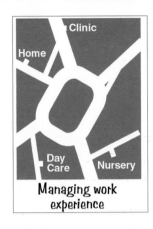

Managing work experience

Experience in the workplace is a valuable part of a vocational health and social care course. Although it is not a compulsory requirement of the Vocational GCSE in Health and Social Care, some schools and colleges may offer a work experience placement as part of the course or as part of the National Curriculum programme of study for Citizenship. At a work experience placement students can develop and practise useful skills, such as **communication** or the **assessment of clients' needs**. Workplace experience can be included in records of achievement, offered as evidence for the Key Skills Qualification and described in job or higher education applications.

Most important of all, students have a chance to find out at first hand about the career path they are interested in and whether, in the end, it is really what they would like to do.

## Finding a placement

Find out, at the beginning of your course, whether or not your school or college will offer to arrange a work placement for you. If not, you may wish to consider arranging your own relevant work experience, perhaps on a part-time basis or during holidays. If your school or college arranges the placement, they may still be very happy for you to make suggestions of your own about where you would like to work, especially if you have contacts in that workplace and could set up the placement yourself.

It is worth bearing in mind that it is often very difficult for teachers and lecturers to find enough suitable placements for their students. Other trainees on professional courses, such as social workers, teachers and nurses, are often given priority for placements. There are also some workplaces where it would not be safe or advisable to offer experience to younger or less qualified students. Therefore, the more active you are in working with your teachers to find your own placements, the more likely you are to work somewhere of direct relevance and benefit to you.

Use your *Yellow Pages*, library and Citizen's Advice Bureau for names, addresses and telephone numbers of workplaces and organisations within a reasonable travelling distance of where you live. Look for:

- hospitals (think about which **areas** of hospital work would be more likely to offer placements)
- community health clinics
- Social Services
- Citizen's Advice Bureaux
- public health authorities
- voluntary agencies
- nurseries and play groups
- schools (including special schools, day or residential)
- probation hostels
- day care centres for people with physical or learning disabilities
- residential homes for people with physical or learning disabilities
- day centres for older people
- residential homes for elders
- complementary health practitioners such as osteopaths, chiropaths and homeopaths
- physiotherapists and occupational therapists.

## Planning the work placement

If you can, try to visit the establishment at which you will be working before the placement begins. Permission to visit may be arranged by your teachers or you may be expected to arrange this yourself. Permission to visit can be requested by telephone or letter. Be willing to give a short description of your course, your intended career and what you hope to achieve from the placement.

Confirm in writing the date and time of your preliminary visit. Once this is arranged, use this opportunity to meet the staff and find out:

- how to get there: routes and travel times
- which key staff you will be working with (try to note down their names)
- the hours you will be working
- the likely tasks you will be involved in
- what type of dress will be suitable
- practical arrangements, for example, where and for how long you will have a lunch break

If you are basing all or part of an assignment on the work placement, take a copy of this and explain the assessment procedure to the person supervising you at the placement. Check with your school or college that the **necessary insurance** has been arranged. This is especially important if you have set up your own placement.

# Making the most of the placement

Many workers in the caring professions are under a great deal of pressure, sometimes because of under-staffing and sometimes because of the nature of the job. It may be an added pressure to work with a student. If you observe the following points it will help your working relationship to flourish.

▶ Find out as much as you can about the placement before you arrive.

▶ Be punctual.

▶ Inform your college/school tutor and your work experience supervisor of any unavoidable absences, but keep these to an absolute minimum.

▶ Be prepared to work different hours from your usual school/college routine.

▶ Be co-operative, friendly and helpful. If there does not seem to be much for you to do, find a moment to ask if you can be given any extra jobs. Use every opportunity to communicate with the patients, clients or service users.

▶ Treat patients, clients or service users with respect.

▶ Observe confidentiality.

▶ Show interest by asking questions at convenient times.

Remember!

The impression you give may affect the employer's willingness to offer placements to students in the future. It is sometimes the case that, following the placement, students are offered further part-time paid work or can even find they return, in the future, for an interview for a full-time post.

## Tasks to be carried out prior to placement

To gain the maximum benefit from the work placement it is vital to be well prepared. The following tasks are suggestions to help you with this preparation.

# Activity

Use the *Skills checklist* (Table 1.12) to carry out a self-appraisal. If there are any areas identified which you feel might cause you problems at the workplace, make sure that you discuss these with your teachers/tutors so that you can plan strategies for dealing with them before the placement begins.

The *Skills checklist* can be used for self-appraisal before and after a work placement. Score 4 for very good, 3 for good, 2 for acceptable and 1 for poor levels of skill.

1. Following your preliminary visit, discuss your feelings and reactions with your teachers, tutors and fellow students. The following areas should be covered:
   - your initial impressions
   - the atmosphere at the placement
   - the patients, clients or service users
   - the staff
   - issues of confidentiality.

2. What you think you will give to and gain from the placement, including how you think the placement could help you acquire the practical and personal skills that you will need in the career you want to follow.

3. It is quite likely that you already have many positive attributes and skills to offer to the placement. It is important to recognise and be proud of these accomplishments. The ways in which you subsequently develop and add to your **skills profile** at the work placement can then be noted. This will give you valuable information to include in a curriculum vitae or future application for a job, training or education.

| SKILL | SCORE | 1 | 2 | 3 | 4 |
|---|---|---|---|---|---|
| Ability to respond to instructions. | | | | | |
| Ability to assess when to ask for help. | | | | | |
| Listening skills. | | | | | |
| Ability to take the initiative. | | | | | |
| Ability to work collaboratively. | | | | | |
| Ability to establish relationships. | | | | | |
| Accuracy in practical tasks. | | | | | |
| Good record of punctuality. | | | | | |
| Time management. | | | | | |
| Ability to respond to criticism. | | | | | |
| Ability to present written reports. | | | | | |
| Ability to handle calculations. | | | | | |
| Good attendance record. | | | | | |
| Ability to show enthusiasm and effort. | | | | | |
| Self-confidence. | | | | | |
| Research skills. | | | | | |

*Table 1.12 Skills checklist for work experience placements*

## Tasks to be carried out in the workplace

Exactly how you use your work experience will depend partly upon the ways you may be using it to write an assignment, write case studies or complete a research project. The following written tasks may help you focus on the kinds of information and experience the placement could offer.

1. Keep a diary or logbook. In it:

   ▶ Note activities undertaken each day and the time spent on them.

   ▶ Record your feelings and reactions to your experiences.

   ▶ Describe the service(s) provided by your work experience establishment. Is there a hierarchical management or staffing structure? Are there different departments? How do the different departments or groups of staff liase with each other?

   ▶ Describe the needs of patients, clients and service users and how they are met.

   ▶ Describe the work of the staff with whom you come into contact. What are the main qualities/skills they need for their jobs? What qualifications and experience do they have?

2. If you hope to use the placement to carry out one or more case studies, you should do so only after a preliminary discussion with placement staff regarding what aspects of the task may be permissible and possible. Confidentiality and respect for the individual, family or group concerned should be maintained. If permission for the study is given, you could do the following.

   ▶ Use your diary or logbook to gather details (such as age, sex, family situation, special interests and abilities, past and current experiences) relevant to the individual(s) or group being studied. Please note that you should never use real names. Use pseudonyms.

   ▶ Analyse the role of the institution or service provider in relation to the individual(s) or group being studied.

   ▶ Make notes on the attitudes and feelings that the patients, clients or service users have towards their situation. Reassure the service user that no real names will be used in your notes.

   ▶ Observe the ways in which staff interact with and influence the patients, clients or service users.

   ▶ Examine and record examples of group interactions and dynamics.

3. Investigate and comment on the following aspects of health and safety in your workplace:

 ▶ safety policy and the role and training of first-aiders.

 ▶ any actual or potential hazards to staff and patients/clients or service users.

 ▶ any provision of rest or reception areas for patients, clients or service users.

4. Evaluate the role of information and communication technologies in the workplace: how they are used, the tasks they are used to perform, and the software employed. Can staff use computers for tasks such as filing and report writing? Assess the potential and actual value of computers and other communication technologies in the workplace.

5. Keep a note in your diary or logbook of any issues or questions arising during the work placement that you would like to discuss with your tutor or other students.

## Tasks to be carried out following the placement

1. Produce an assessment of your strengths and weaknesses during your placement. Refer back to your **skills checklist** completed prior to the placement.

 ▶ Has your self-appraisal changed?

 ▶ Have your career aims changed?

 ▶ Have you gained additional skills useful for your intended career? Update your curriculum vitae and, if possible, plan strategies for overcoming any remaining areas of weakness or skills gaps.

2. Give an oral presentation describing your work experience to other students. This should include:

 ▶ your own role and tasks – what you were expected to do

 ▶ the challenges and problems you faced

 ▶ an assessment of what you have learned and what personal development you feel has taken place.

3. Try to ensure that you have a chance to talk informally to your tutors and teachers about the placement. You should also have the chance to receive more formal assessment and feedback on your work from your placement supervisor, your tutor/teachers and your fellow students.

4. Write a letter of thanks to the employer(s) concerned.

5. Prepare a written evaluation of the placement.

   ▶ What aspects were the most or least satisfactory?

   ▶ What changes would you make in the workplace if you could?
   Give reasons.

   ▶ Would you recommend the placement to another student?

# RESOURCES

## Books

Buzan, T. (1993), *The Mind Map Book*. London, BBC Publications.

Buzan, T. (1995), *Use Your Memory*. London, BBC Books.

Buzan, T (1996), *Use Your Head*. London, BBC Books.

Cardwell, M (1996), *The Complete A–Z Psychology Handbook*. London, Hodder and Stoughton.

Gilroy, D.E. and Miles, TR. (1996) *Dyslexia at College*. Routledge.

Indge, B. (1997) *The Complete A–Z Biology Handbook*. London, Hodder and Stougton.

Lawson, T. and Garrod, J. (1996), *The Complete A–Z Sociology Handbook*. London, Hodder and Stoughton.

Mitchell, J.E. (1998), *Student Organiser Pack*, London: Communication and Learning Skills Centre, 131 Homefield Park, Sutton, Surrey, SMI 2DY.

Nortledge, A. (1990) *The Good Study Guide*. Milton Keynes, The Open University.

Richards, J. (1999) *The Complete A–Z Health and Social Care Handbook*. London, Hodder and Stoughton.

## Software

*Type to Learn* (Windows, Mac) – teaches students to type while reinforcing spelling, grammar, composition and punctuation skills. Available from Iansyst Tel: 01223 420101

*Touch-type, read and spell* – specially designed for dyslexic learners by Philip Alexandre Tel: 0181 464 1330.

*Touch Type* (Windows, Acorn, Mac) see, hear, type from Inclusive Technology Tel: 01457 81970.

*Mavis Beacon Teaches Typing* – Mindscape. Version 8 English. Available from most high streets stores or Priority House, Charles Av, Maltings Park, Burgess Hill, W. Sussex RH15 9TQ

*Wordswork for Windows* 3.x/95/98/NT – cost for single person's use £125.00 Distributed by iANSYST Ltd and Brind Arena/Ellen Morgan. Enquiries to sales@dyslexic.com or phone 01223 420101.

Aimed at dyslexic undergraduates, this programme is also useful for students in upper secondary, tertiary and further education and for dyslexic adults wanting to improve their skills before returning to formal study. The programme uses graphics, voice-overs, colour and humour to develop language skills in essay writing, revision, grammar, handwriting, memory, oral presentation, punctuation, reading, spelling, time management and vocabulary building.

*textHELP! Read and Write* for Windows 5 – cost £115 + VAT.
Distributed by iANSYST Ltd. FREEphone 08000 1800 45
The White House,
72 Fen Road,
Cambridge CB4 1UN
Tel 01223 420101 Fax: 01223 42 66 44
sales@dyslexic.com  website – www.dyslexic.com

This programme includes an advanced phonetic spell checker, a word prediction facility, homophone support and a log which will record typical spelling errors for future analysis.

*Dyslexia and ICT – Building on Success* by Sally McKeown (Becta Publications 2000, Becta Bookshop, Milburn Hill Road, Science Park, Coventry CV4 7BR) is a very useful guide to software for dyslexic students.

## Organisations

British Dyslexia Association
98 London Rd,
Reading RG1 5AU
Helpline 0118 966 8271, Administration 0118 966 2677
email – info@dyslexia.demon.co.uk
website – www.bda-dyslexia.org.uk

The Dyspraxia Foundation,
8, West Alley,
Hitchin, Herts SG5 IEG
Helpline: 01462 454986

Skill (National Bureau for Students with Disabilities)
3rd Floor,
Chapter House,
18–20 Crucifix Lane,
London SE1 3JW
Tel. 0800 3285050

Royal National Institute for the Deaf (RNID)
19–23 Featherstone St.
London ECIY 8SL
Helpline – freephone 0808 808 0123, textphone 0870 6033 007
email – informationline@rnid.org.uk
website – www.rnid.org.uk

Royal National Institute for the Blind (RNIB)
224 Great Portland Street
London WIN 6AA
Helpline – 0845 766 999
Customer services Tel: 0845 702 3153
Textphone: 0800 515152
website – www.rnib.org.uk

Disablement Information and Advice Lines (DIAL UK)
Park Lodge,
St. Catherine's Hospital
Tickhill Road,
Balby, Doncaster
South Yorkshire DN4 8QN
01302 310123

## Other

Students with dyslexia, dyspraxia or other disability in full time education may be able to claim a **Disabled Students Allowance**. This is a lump sum with which the student can pay for equipment or services, e.g. to buy a tape recorder and/or photocopying and specialist tuition. For more information about this allowance contact your local Education Authority (if you live in England) and ask for an application form for the allowance. If your school or college has a disability co-ordinator, she or he should also be able to help and advise on how to make a claim.

# Glossary

**action plan**
a detailed and structured plan for an assignment or piece of work.

**analyse**
examine in detail: separate into component parts.

**assignments**
pieces of work set and assessed as part of the requirements of the course.

**autonomous learners**
students who have become self-reliant.

**bibliography**
a list of the books referred to in an assignment, essay or other piece.

**brainstorming**
a way of generating ideas before beginning a piece of work.

**client**
an individual receiving support, treatment or therapy from a health or social care service.

**comparison**
an analysis of similarities and differences.

**conclusion**
a summing up, for example, of ideas, arguments or evidence used in an assignment or essay.

**confidentiality**
respect for the privacy of any information about a client. It is one of the principles which underpins all health and social care practice.

**critical evaluation**
where evidence has been used to support judgements or views.

**cueing and signal words**
words which, in a written or oral presentation, warn of impending and significant changes in the pace, emphasis and order of the content.

**curriculum vitae CV**
a brief account of one's education and previous occupation often required when applying for a new job.

**define**
give an exact meaning of a word or concept.

**describe**
give a written, visual or oral account, as required.

**discuss**
consider an issue from various points of view.

**dyslexia**
dyslexia is evident when fluent and accurate word identification (reading) and/or spelling is learnt very incompletely or with great difficulty.

**editing**
checking a document for errors/making changes or modifications.

**evaluation**
a retrospective review or reassessment.

**feedback**
to 'give feedback' has come to mean to make a formal or semiformal response to a piece of work or action.

**grading requirements**
the criteria which determine the grades awarded for the course.

**ICT**
Information and Communication Technologies i.e. the use of the Internet or Intra net systems as well as computers, Dictaphones, tape recorders, word processors, hardware and software programs, voice mall, fax, E-mail, CD ROM, telephones, electronic spell checkers etc.

**identify**
pick out key characteristics or what is most important.

**illustrate**
give examples to support points made.

**Internet**
an international computer network linking computers from educational institutions, government agencies, industry and domestic users etc.

**interpret**
show or make clear the meaning.

**introduction**
a preliminary section at the beginning of a book or piece of work.

**justify**
show good reasons for.

**meta cognition**
the ability to 'think about thinking'.

**mind-mapping**
a technique used to organise thoughts and ideas in linked key words and pictures. This method can be used for generating ideas and planning work as well as note-taking and revising.

**mnemonic**
a device which aids the memory.

**motivation**
to be stimulated by or interested in something.

**multisensory**
methods of learning which simultaneously 'tap' more than one sense.

**note-taking**
a way of summarising points in a text which are relevant to whatever is being studied.

**personal organisation**
refers to the ways in which an individual plans and manages their daily responsibilities.

**portfolio**
a collection of the different types of evidence which can show successful completion of the course.

**primary sources**
information or data gathered at first hand.

**prioritising**
putting things in order of importance so that the most pressing issues are tackled first.

**proof**
evidence that something is 'true'.

**proofreading**
reading through a document for errors.

**PQ4R**
a reading and note-taking method: **P**review, **Q**uestion, **R**ead, **R**eflect, **R**ecite, **R**eview.

**reception reading**
where reading takes place at a steady pace and what is being read is fairly easy to absorb and understand.

**records of achievement**
a portfolio of educational and personal achievement.

**reflective reading**
reading which involves thinking about and evaluating what is read.

**secondary sources**
information or data from the work or research of other people.

**service user**
an individual using or accessing a social or public service.

**skim-reading**
the process of running eyes over a text to extract essential or key information.

**special assessment concessions**
special test arrangements (such as extra time) and/or special consideration (action taken after the examination) in public examinations.

**spell-checker**
an electronic dictionary.

**spider diagrams**
a diagrammatic way of representing ideas or information which brings out the main themes and their relationships to each other.

**theory**
a system of ideas explaining something.

**thesaurus**
a book that lists words in groups of synonyms (words with similar meanings) and related concepts.

**visual thinker**
someone who prefers to organise their thoughts in images or patterns.

**work experience**
time spent in a workplace to gain related experience and knowledge.

# Health, social care and early years provision

## CHAPTER CONTENT

This chapter will help you learn about:

▶ the range of needs of major client groups

▶ the types of services that exist to meet client group needs and how they are organised

▶ the ways people can obtain care services and the barriers that can prevent people from gaining access to services

▶ the main work roles and skills of people who provide health, social care and early years services

▶ the values that underpin all care work with clients.

You will understand more about the work of health, social care and early years service providers by:

▶ understanding how services are developed in response to social policy goals and to meet the needs of individuals

▶ knowing about the different services and job roles.

**Unit 1, Health, social care and early years provision** is assessed through your portfolio work. Your overall result for the unit will be a grade on the scale from G to A*.

In each section of this chapter, you will find exercises and activities to help you work through the material. At the end of the chapter, you will find a list of key words, references used in the chapter, lists of useful addresses and possible resources you or your teacher could find helpful.

Answers to activities, where appropriate, can be found at the end of the chapter.

# THE CARE NEEDS OF MAJOR CLIENT GROUPS

In this section we will look at the **differing needs of major client groups** and how services are designed to meet these needs.

Needs can be separated into three areas:

▶ health needs

▶ developmental needs

▶ social care needs.

Table 2.1 shows examples of how these needs could be grouped under these different categories.

| HEALTH NEEDS | DEVELOPMENTAL NEEDS | SOCIAL CARE NEEDS |
|---|---|---|
| • Keeping healthy<br>• Freedom from infection<br>• Freedom from disease<br>• Freedom from illness<br>• Good eyesight<br>• Healthy body<br>• Good diet<br>• Exercise<br>• Personal hygiene<br>• Good hearing<br>• Dental health<br>• Screening for disease<br>• Prevention of ill health<br>• Immunisation against disease<br>• Medication to support health<br>• Pollution-free environment | • Language skills<br>• Written skills<br>• Social skills<br>• Developing personal relationships<br>• Making use of one's abilities<br>• Stimulating work<br>• Learning new skills<br>• Leisure activities<br>• Developing and maintaining independence<br>• Developing effective communication | • Emotional support<br>• Adequate clothing shelter, warmth, safe environment, physical support and help<br>• Financial support<br>• Social interaction<br>• Adequate food<br>• Promotion of independence, dignity |

Table 2.1 The needs of clients in health and social care

# Problems with grouping

Very often it can be difficult to decide which need fits into which heading – the need to stay warm can be seen to be a health need (if older people become very cold and develop hypothermia they will need medical treatment), but staying warm could also be seen as a social care need.

At different stages of our lives our needs may change, and the type of support we need may also alter.

In this section we will look in more detail at the needs of the following client groups:

▶ babies and young children

▶ adolescents and young people

▶ adults

▶ older people

▶ people with disabilities.

# Babies

A baby is defined as **aged under one year old**. In the first year of life a baby is very dependent on adults, usually parents, to provide their health, developmental and social care needs. During this first year, a baby develops from being totally dependent to becoming mobile, and developing the ability to interact with others and to play.

## Discussion

### Health needs

You may have included the following in your list:

▶ making sure the baby has the recommended immunisations

▶ keeping the baby away from sources of infection

▶ making sure that feeds and equipment used by the baby are clean.

### Social care needs

You may have included the following in your list:

▶ keeping the baby warm

▶ dressing the baby in adequate clothing.

### Developmental needs

▶ interacting with the baby to encourage development

▶ providing suitable toys and other stimulation.

## Activity

Look at Table 2.1 and identify the key needs that are relevant in the first year of life.
How would you make sure that these needs are met?

## Young children

As children grow older they are able to do more for themselves, but they are still dependent on other people to look after them. Children experience many changes as they grow, going to playgroups, nursery, and infants school. They may have a new brother or sister. They will make friends outside the family and develop new interests and new skills, such as learning to ride a tricycle.

### Discussion

One of the key difficulties facing parents of young children is balancing the need to encourage independence and self-confidence while making sure that risks to the child are reduced. Living with risk is part of life, and if we try to reduce all risk we can affect the positive development of a young child.

### *Health needs*

You may have included in your list immunisations, maintaining a healthy diet and lifestyle, and personal hygiene, such as encouraging children to wash their hands after using the toilet and before eating meals.

### *Developmental needs*

From childhood the development of independence and social relationships is a very important aspect of growing up.

### *Social care needs*

Clothing, a safe environment, and emotional support could be included here.

## Adolescents and young people

Adolescence and the teenage years are seen as a period of rapid growth and development and emotional change.

## Activity

By the age of seven most children have developed a range of skills, including reading and writing, and their language is well established so they are able to communicate their feelings.
Look at Table 2.1 and decide which needs are most relevant to Thomas.

## Activity

Perhaps you are a teenager yourself. If not, imagine being a 14 year old today. Make a list of all the good things about being 14. Then make a list of all the bad things about being 14. You could compare your list with other people in your class. How are they similar and how are they different? Are there differences depending on whether you are a girl or a boy? Some people find that parents are stricter with their daughters than with their sons.

Table 2.2 shows the answers given by youth workers who were given this exercise.

Look at the table, and think about the needs that young people may have as a result of their experience of being 14. Although this can be an exciting time, young people can also experience confusion, sadness and anxiety.

Look at Table 2.1 again, and identify the different needs that this age group may have. The family may not be able to meet all the needs of this age group. Other health and care workers may need to be involved in supporting them. These could include school nurses, specialist workers dealing with drugs, sexual health and mental health problems.

**Connexions** is a government programme aimed at meeting the needs of young people between the age of 13 and 19 as they approach adulthood.

**Table 2.2 Experience of being 14 years old**

| POSITIVE | NEGATIVE |
|---|---|
| ● Meeting new people | ● Feeling shy and awkward, meeting new people |
| ● Trying out new experiences:<br>  – drinking alcohol<br>  – smoking<br>  – going out with friends<br>  – belonging to a group | ● Having spots/weight problems<br>● Starting periods/voice breaking<br>● Physical changes: breasts, body hair |
| ● More personal freedom | ● Feeling lonely, isolated |
| ● Having first girlfriend/boyfriend | ● Parents don't understand you |
| ● Trying out new clothes, hairstyles, make-up | ● Not belonging to a group |
| ● Having first job – earning money | ● Worried about school work, bullying |
| ● Feeling grown up | ● Not having a girlfriend/boyfiend |
| ● Feeling independent | ● Anxiety about sexuality |
| ● Deciding what to do in free time | ● Being treated like a child |
| ● Close friendships | ● Too young to do some things, too old to do others |
| ● Excited about the future | ● Trouble with police, teachers |
| ● Sense of personal identity | ● Anxiety about the opposite sex |
| | ● Dislike of own appearance |
| | ● Using drugs, sniffing glue, getting drunk as a way of coping |
| | ● Depressed and anxious about the future |
| | ● Not sure of own identity |

# Activity

Go to the Connexions website: www.connexions.gov.uk and look at the services provided. There will be a local service in your area. You should be able to find details about it in your school, youth club or library.

## Adults

Becoming adult does not mean that we no longer have needs. Adults may have greater pressures put on them through work and family responsibilities, including the care of young and older family members. There can be additional pressures because of gender stereotyping, with women being seen as the natural carers in the family, although they may also be working, and men still being seen as the main breadwinner of the family, in spite of rising unemployment in traditional male jobs.

## CASE STUDY TWO: MARCELLA

Marcella is a single parent of 35. She has two children, a boy aged eight and a girl aged 10, who are collected from school by a childminder who looks after them until Marcella finishes work. Marcella works in the housing department of the local council, where she helps find accommodation for homeless families. The job is stressful, and often Marcella does not have a lunch break as she tries to keep up to date with all the paperwork. On her way home, she shops in the local supermarket, preparing a quick meal after she has collected the children. Marcella is too tired to go out in the evening, although sometimes she has to drive the children to a swimming club or other activity. Because she is always in a hurry, Marcella drives to and from work, and she has little exercise during the day. At her last medical check up, the practice nurse noted that she had put on weight and her blood pressure was higher than it should be for her age.

▶ What are Marcella's needs? How could these needs be met?

▶ How may Marcella's needs change as she gets older, for example when she reaches 45 years old and then when she reaches 60 years old?

## Older people

Statistics show that more people are living into their eighties and nineties, and this client group may have particular needs. Physical ageing is a natural process and can result in declining physical ability, including loss of vision, and hearing and mobility problems.

CASE STUDY
THREE:
BEATRICE

Beatrice is 90 years old, she is a widow and lives on her own in a three-bedroomed house. Her married daughter sees her every week. Beatrice has diabetes, and this has caused problems with her sight and also with ulcers on her leg. The local social services have organised a home help who comes weekly to clean the house; a shopper comes every fortnight to do her shopping. Beatrice is very independent and, although she has problems walking because of arthritis, she gets the local minibus service to the town once a week to collect her pension. Beatrice enjoys reading, but listening to the radio and watching television are becoming more difficult as she is quite deaf. Many of her friends have died, and she has no contact with her neighbours.

▶ What are Beatrice's needs? Can you group them under the headings used in Table 2.1?

▶ Who can support Beatrice so that she can fulfil these needs?

## Discussion

Although Beatrice has some clearly identified health needs, such as the need to monitor her diabetes, we can see that her health needs have an impact on all aspects of her life. If Beatrice cannot communicate easily because of her hearing problem, and cannot get out and about because of the arthritis, this affects her development and her ability to interact with others and to lead a fulfilling life. Many older people are not aware of financial benefits they are entitled to, and this can affect their health and social care needs, as they are worried about not being able to pay for heating and other bills so they do not eat properly or keep warm.

## Disabled people

People with disabilities make up about 14% of the population aged 16+ according to the 1991 census figures. Disabilities can include:

▶ sensory disabilities – hearing, vision

▶ physical disabilities, which may affect mobility, and could include cerebral palsy

▶ mental health problems, such as schizophrenia or depression

▶ learning disabilities, such as Downs Syndrome.

Some disabilities are inherited conditions, such as Huntingtons Chorea, where a faulty gene leads to the disabling condition.

Some disabilities are developmental conditions, where the foetus is affected in the womb in some way, such as if the mother contracts Rubella (German measles), and this can cause deafness and blindness.

Illness and accident are the main causes of disability occurring in those born without a disability. Road traffic accidents are the most common cause of accidents causing disability.

In this section we have looked at different client groups and identified their needs.

## CASE STUDY FOUR:

Look at the following examples of disabled clients and decide what health, social care and developmental needs they have.

1. Vikram is a 20-year-old student with cerebral palsy. He has normal intelligence but he has a problem with mobility and speech. He finds it difficult to walk long distances. He is following a full-time course at a local college. He finds it difficult to make friends.

2. Jessica is four years old. She has Downs Syndrome. At the moment she is in a nursery class attached to a mainstream infants school. Jessica is very active and needs constant supervision. Her parents want her to go to the infants school, but the teachers feel her needs will be met more effectively in a Special School. Jessica's speech and writing skills are slow to develop, although she is able to use the toilet and feed herself. Other children in the class tend to avoid her.

3. Mark is 26. He had a car accident when he was 18. He is a wheelchair user. At the moment he works in the office of a charity for disabled people as a fundraiser. He wants to move to a flat and be independent. He has an adapted car. He can manage his own personal care, but needs help with housework and shopping.

4. Ted is 55. When he was 40 he travelled abroad for his company. He contracted a rare virus which left him paralysed from the neck down. He has regained some use in his arms and can feed himself, but he is dependent on others for his personal care and transport. He lives at home with his wife. The house has been adapted. He has to be careful to avoid coughs and colds as these can have a serious effect on his lungs. He spends a lot of time advising other disabled people and being involved in several voluntary groups.

We can see from these examples that we cannot lump all disabled people together. They are all individuals, and their needs differ according to their age and personality as well as their individual disability.

Some of these needs may be met by the family members or by the individual themselves. However, additional support may sometimes be needed from other health and social care workers.

Figure 2.1 shows the different workers that may be involved in the different client groups. We will look at the roles of these workers later in this chapter.

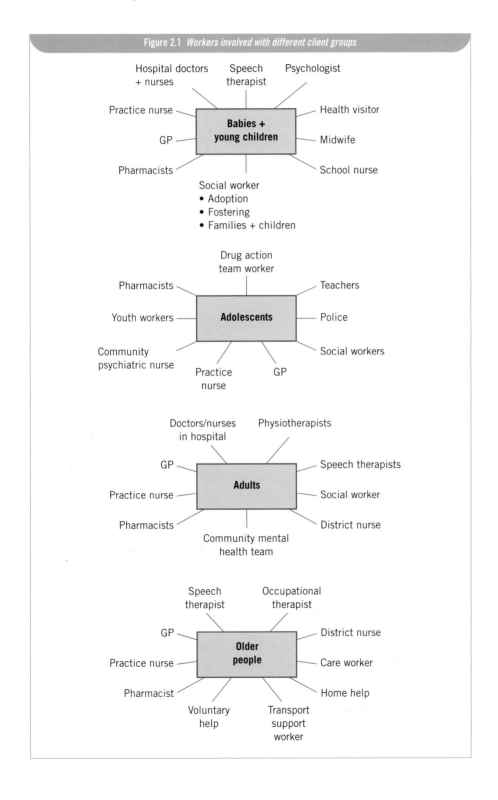

**Figure 2.1 Workers involved with different client groups**

# KEY SOCIAL POLICY IN THE 21ST CENTURY

Social policy is about the government's plans to provide services in the following key areas:

▶ education

▶ housing

▶ income management (either through benefits or earned income)

▶ health services

▶ social services.

Social policy is affected by certain factors (see Figure 2.2).

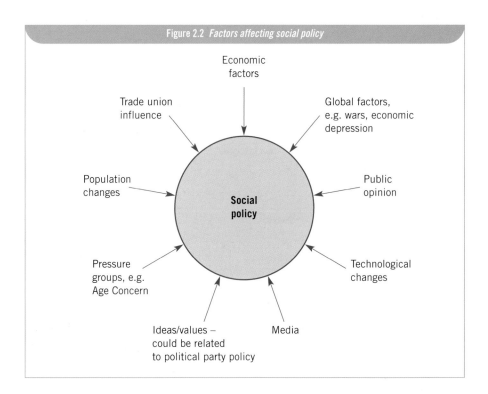

Figure 2.2 *Factors affecting social policy*

Economic factors

Trade union influence

Global factors, e.g. wars, economic depression

Population changes

**Social policy**

Public opinion

Pressure groups, e.g. Age Concern

Technological changes

Ideas/values – could be related to political party policy

Media

## Identifying needs

Different regions of the UK have different needs. The local health authorities identify the needs of their population and then develop services to meet those needs. At the same time, national priorities are identified in health care, and national programmes are also introduced.

Examples of local health programmes to meet local needs:

▶ sexual health clinics aimed at young people, and contraceptive advice and support are offered in an area that has a high teenage pregnancy rate

▶ diabetes support clinics are specifically provided for women from Asian backgrounds who are more likely to have diabetes

Some of these programmes may be part of national schemes like the Health Action Zones.

Examples of national health programmes to meet national needs:

▶ stop smoking programmes that have been developed locally as part of the national programme to reduce the numbers of people smoking

▶ National Service Frameworks in Coronary Heart Disease and Mental Health, which have been developed in response to the evidence of the need to reduce heart disease and suicide (*Saving Lives, Our Healthier Nation*, 1999).

In all these programmes, statistics such as causes of death and incidence of disease are collected, and the health needs of the population identified and plans are made to improve health.

Each year the District Health Authority produces a report. In this report the identified needs of the area are reported and the plans to meet these needs are outlined. The Health Authority may identify needs in a variety of ways, through questionnaires, public meetings, group meetings, etc. This process is called a **health needs assessment**, and is usually led by the Public Health Unit. Figure 2.3 shows an example of profiling a community to identify needs.

The local council does a similar exercise to establish needs for housing, transport and social care needs. Many of these exercises focus on the needs of particular groups, such as older people, disabled groups and children.

The government also has its own websites that give information about proposed health and social care services. These are given at the end of the chapter.

## Activity

Copies of health needs assessments and of **community plans** are often available in libraries, or direct from the Health Authority or Council. Many of these organisations have their own websites which give details of services planned for the future. See if you can find your local websites.

**mortality rates** – death rates
**morbidity rates** – stastistics showing the level of illness in the population
**epidemiology** – the study of the rates of disease

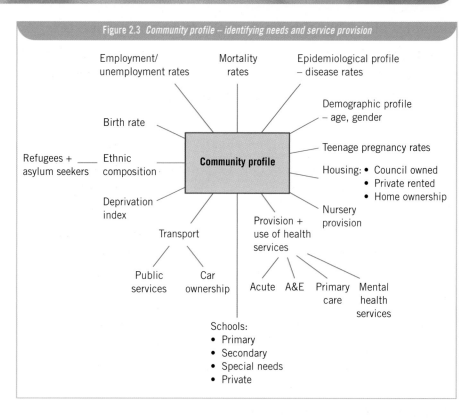

Figure 2.3 *Community profile – identifying needs and service provision*

As we can see from these examples, needs are identified and services are then developed to meet these needs.

## Population changes

When planning housing, education and health and care services, population changes have to be identified.

In the UK, the population is becoming increasingly older, with people living longer and having fewer children (a reduced birth rate). Current predictions for population changes in the 21st century include an increase in the number of people aged over 65 and a reduction in the 25 to 45 age group.

In your groups, discuss what effect this will have on the five key social policy areas.

### Discussion

*Education*

If there is a reduction in adults of working age, there may be difficulties in recruiting teachers. We have already seen that the national shortage of teachers has led to schools recruiting staff from abroad.

### Housing

With more older people living longer, more sheltered housing will be needed. Because women tend to outlive men and live on their own, the numbers of single households will increase.

### Income management

If there are fewer people of working age, the government will not be able to raise money through direct taxation and national insurance on people's wages. This money goes towards benefits and pensions. If there are increased numbers of people over pensionable age, more pensions will be paid by the State. The government is already trying to deal with this problem by raising the retirement age for women to 65 and by encouraging people to buy their own pensions.

### Health services

People over 65 make more use of the health service, and if this group increases, more services will be needed, such as chiropody, physiotherapy, and surgery for cataracts and joint replacements. However, if the work force declines there will be a problem having enough staff to meet the increased demand.

### Social services

People over 65 make more use of social services. Because of the possible shortage of staff, alternatives to day centres, residential homes and other services will be considered. Clients will be encouraged to stay independently in their own homes for as long as possible.

We have seen that services are developed and provided to meet changing situations. We will now look at specific areas of social policy that are seen to be a key target for the 21st century.

# Child poverty

Poverty is difficult to define. Within the European Union the poverty line is usually drawn at below 50% of the average income in that particular society. In the past what was called **National Assistance** (benefits paid by the State) was based on the minimum level of income required to sustain life. This amount was criticised as it meant that no-one could do anything else but exist on this amount – no birthday cards or presents, no holidays and no social activity, including using transport, was possible. In the UK in 2002, poverty is defined as households that have an income below 60% of the average median income.

**The median average** is the figure that occurs in the middle of the range of incomes. If we used the **arithmetic mean** as an average, this could give an incorrect idea of the average as it would include very high earners, and this would inflate the overall average.

## Activity

Study Table 2.3 and identify the patterns you see.
Which groups are most likely to be in poverty?

Table 2.3 shows households that have an income below 60% of the median income.

| United Kingdom and Great Britain[1] | | | Percentages | |
|---|---|---|---|---|
| | 1981 | 1991–92 | 1996–97 | 1998–99 |
| Head or spouse unemployed | 52 | 71 | 62 | 64 |
| Head or spouse aged 60 or over | 19 | 31 | 24 | 26 |
| One or more in part-time work | 24 | 26 | 25 | 24 |
| Self-employed[2] | 13 | 19 | 19 | 20 |
| One in full-time work, one not working | 8 | 12 | 15 | 14 |
| One in full-time, one in part-time work | 2 | 3 | 3 | 4 |
| Single or couple, all in full-time work | 1 | 2 | 2 | 2 |
| Other[3] | 36 | 51 | 42 | 41 |
| All | 13 | 21 | 18 | 18 |

[1] Data for 1981 and 1991–92 are based on the Family Expenditure Survey which covers the United Kingdom. Data for 1996–97 and 1998–99 are based on the Family Resources Survey which covers Great Britain only.

[2] Those in benefit units which contain one or more adults who are normally self-employed for 31 or more hours a week.

[3] Includes long-term sick and disabled people and non-working single-parents.

Source: Social Trends 2001, HMSO

Table 2.3 Individuals in housholds with incomes below 60% of median income

In 2001 the government aims were to reduce the number of children living in low income families by a quarter by 2004, by a half by 2010 and totally by 2020.

We can see from Figure 2.4 that children are present in many households with low incomes. Twenty-four per cent of children (or 3.1 million) were living in such households in 1998/9 in Great Britain. In 1991/2 and 1992/3 there were 27% of children living in poverty.

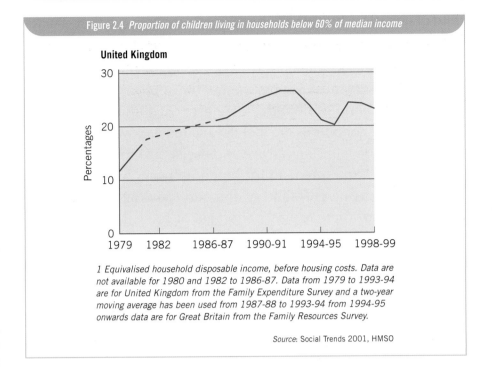

Figure 2.4 *Proportion of children living in households below 60% of median income*

1 Equivalised household disposable income, before housing costs. Data are not available for 1980 and 1982 to 1986-87. Data from 1979 to 1993-94 are for United Kingdom from the Family Expenditure Survey and a two-year moving average has been used from 1987-88 to 1993-94 from 1994-95 onwards data are for Great Britain from the Family Resources Survey.

*Source*: Social Trends 2001, HMSO

## What is the government planning to do?

▶ The 1999 *Working Families Tax Credit* guarantees a minimum income of £214 per week for families who are working who have young children.

▶ Lone parents tend to be in poverty. The government's *New Deal* offers a programme for lone parents to return to work and gives financial help towards the cost of child care.

▶ The *Early Years Child Care Partnership* is another initiative that is being developed nationally and locally to support working parents by offering child care.

▶ *Sure Start* programmes include payments to mothers of young children.

▶ A range of other benefits are being developed to assist parents of young children. The details are given in the following booklets: *Babies and Children* BC1, *Expecting a baby* BC2, *Bringing up Children* BC3, *New Deal for Lone Parents* LP 15.

## Homelessness

Since 1982 there has been an increase in homelessness in Great Britain. In Wales, three out of 10 households accepted as homeless in 1999 stated that they were homeless as a result of a breakdown of a relationship with a partner. In Scotland, almost a

# Activity

You should be able to find these leaflets in the library or post office. When you find them, look through them and make a list of all the benefits and support that is available to parents of children.

## Activity

Figure 2.5 shows the numbers of households in temporary accommodation between 1982 and 1999. Look at the figure and describe the main patterns you see.

## Activity

What are the main problems that rough sleepers may experience?

third of homeless households were homeless because they did not wish to remain with friends or family.

When a homeless household makes an application, the local housing authority must decide whether the applicant is eligible for assistance, is unintentionally homeless, or is in a priority need group. If these conditions are met in England and Wales, the council must provide sufficient advice and assistance to the applicant. In England the main reason for homelessness is related to the increase in housing costs in London and the South East, and to asylum seekers. There is also a shortage of council housing available to rent. Across Great Britain, one in seven households in temporary accommodation were housed in hostels (including womens refuges) and one in seven were in bed and breakfast accommodation. The Rough Sleepers Unit (RSU) was set up in 1999 as part of the government's Social Exclusion Policy of 1998. By June 2000, the number of people sleeping rough in England on any one night was estimated to be about 1.2. million.

### Discussion

Homeless people tend to have a shorter life expectancy. Because they have no fixed address, they have difficulty accessing benefits, obtaining work and being registered with a doctor.

What do you think the government should do about homeless people?

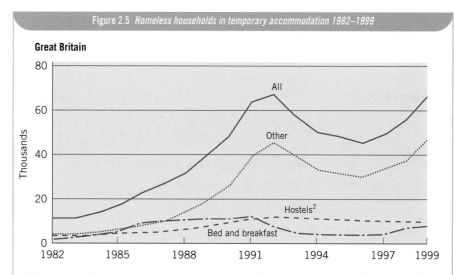

**Figure 2.5** *Homeless households in temporary accommodation 1982–1999*

1 Data are at end year and include households awaiting the outcome of homeless enquries. Households made temporarily homeless through flooding in Wales in 1990 and 1993 are excluded.
2 From 1987 the data for Wales include those households placed in women's refuges.

*Source:* Social Trends 2001, HMSO

# Drug misuse

Drug misuse is associated with poor health, both directly, for example through the effects of overdoses and the spread of infection (specifically HIV/AIDS and hepatitis B and C), and indirectly, because of the link with social exclusion through homelessness, poverty, unemployment and criminal behaviour. In *Tackling Drugs to Build a Better Britain* (HMSO 1998) the government decided to adopt an approach that would focus on prevention and treatment of drug misuse. The aims of the programme against drug misuse were to:

▶ help young people resist drug misuse

▶ protect local communities from drug-related anti-social and criminal behaviour

▶ enable people with drug-related problems to overcome them and live healthy crime-free lives

▶ reduce the availability of illegal drugs.

Local councils worked with local primary care groups to develop action plans against drug misuse. These are some of the ways in which one local group developed a strategy against drugs in their local area.

1. To work closely with the police so that young people who are arrested for drug misuse are offered support and treatment.

2. To introduce the Healthy Schools programme into all secondary schools.

3. To provide a young people's community worker, who will visit youth clubs and other key meeting places.

4. To target habitual drug offenders and encourage them to seek treatment.

**Table 2.4 Percentage of people who had used certain drugs in the last year, 1998**

| England & Wales | 16–19 | 20–24 | Percentages All aged 16–24 |
|---|---|---|---|
| Cannabis | 28 | 26 | 27 |
| Amphetamine | 9 | 10 | 10 |
| Ecstasy | 4 | 6 | 5 |
| Poppers | 4 | 5 | 5 |
| Magic mushrooms | 4 | 3 | 4 |
| Cocaine | 1 | 5 | 3 |
| LSD | 2 | 3 | 3 |
| Any drug | 31 | 28 | 29 |

*Source: Social Trends 2001, HMSO*

# Activity

1. One of the key problems has been to reduce the amount of illicit drug use by 16 to 29 year olds. Table 2.4 shows the numbers of young people estimated to be using illegal drugs. Look at the figures and describe what you see.

2. Many schools have joined the Healthy Schools National Programme, and young people have been given information about the dangers of drug misuse in a variety of ways, including drama groups and projects. Here is a list of ways in which local groups have tried to get the message across to young people. Decide which ways are most effective.

   ▶ Posters
   ▶ Leaflets
   ▶ Talk by a nurse
   ▶ Group work with a youth worker who specialises in working with young drug users
   ▶ Film or video
   ▶ Talk by an ex-drug user
   ▶ Play produced by a local company involving members of the school
   ▶ Talk by a policeman or policewoman to the whole school

3. How would you design an anti-drugs programme in your school or college?

These three examples of social policy (child poverty, homelessness and drug misuse) are being developed in a partnership between the statutory sector (the local council and the health service), the voluntary sector and the private sector. Partnership is one of the key approaches used in all aspects of social policy.

# TYPES OF CARE SERVICES

This section covers the types of care services that are provided to meet the needs of different client groups.

Health, social care services and early years services can be divided into four separate divisions.

▶ statutory
▶ private
▶ voluntary
▶ informal.

1. **Statutory services** are funded and provided by central or local government agencies. Examples of statutory health services are

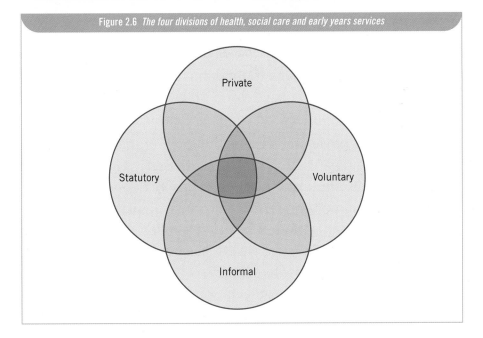

Figure 2.6 *The four divisions of health, social care and early years services*

NHS services, including hospitals, school nursing and commu-nity nursing. Examples of statutory social care services would be the services provided by the local authority social services department.

2. **Private services** provide a range of services, including private hospitals, private residential homes and private nurseries and these are run to make a profit.

3. **Voluntary services** are provided by voluntary (or non-profit making) organisations that are usually registered as charities and may provide services to particular client groups, e.g. Age Concern provides day centres for older people, Mencap pro-vides a range of services to people with learning difficulties.

4. **Informal Services** are provided outside the other three sectors and are usually unpaid. Examples of informal care would be a local church lunch club, a babysitting group, and relatives caring for older family members.

# Activity

Look at the following list and decide whether each service is statutory, voluntary, private or informal.
1. A married daughter looking after her 75-year-old mother
2. A GP (general practitioner or family doctor)
3. A 'Meals on Wheels' service
4. A consultant working in a private hospital

# The national organisation of the NHS

The White Paper, *The New NHS, Modern, Dependable*, was published in 1997 and outlined the plans to modernise the NHS over the next ten years. Many changes have taken place in the organisation of health care, and we will look at some of these in this section.

The Department of Health is the national government department in charge of the organisation of the Health Service in the UK. With the changes that are taking place in Wales, Scotland and Ireland, these regions will be taking over the control of health in their own areas, but the organisation of health is similar in all parts of the UK. The Secretary of State for Health has overall responsibility for the NHS. Do you know his/her name?

Figure 2.7 shows how the NHS is divided into regions.

▶ England is divided into eight regions.

▶ Wales is divided into five regions.

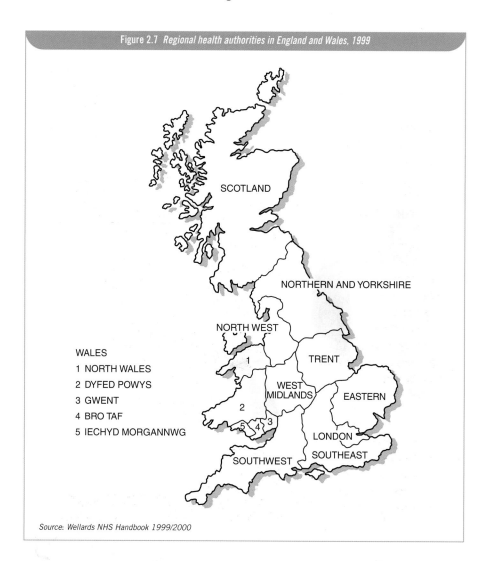

**Figure 2.7  Regional health authorities in England and Wales, 1999**

WALES
1 NORTH WALES
2 DYFED POWYS
3 GWENT
4 BRO TAF
5 IECHYD MORGANNWG

*Source: Wellards NHS Handbook 1999/2000*

▶ Scotland is divided into 15 Health Boards.

▶ Northern Ireland is divided into four Health and Social Care Boards (Figure 2.8).

As you can see the regions are very different. Some areas are highly populated with towns and cities, other regions are in remote rural areas. Each region has a Regional Health Authority that is responsible for the NHS in the region. Each region is further divided into District Health Authorities. Figure 2.9 shows the organisation of the NHS at regional level. The full map of regional and health authorities is available on the following website www.doh.gov.uk/pub/docs/doh/romap.pdf. Using the Internet, see if you can identify your region on it.

From April 2002, there will be further changes to the organisations of the NHS. District Health Authorities will be merged, and will become Strategic Health Authorities.

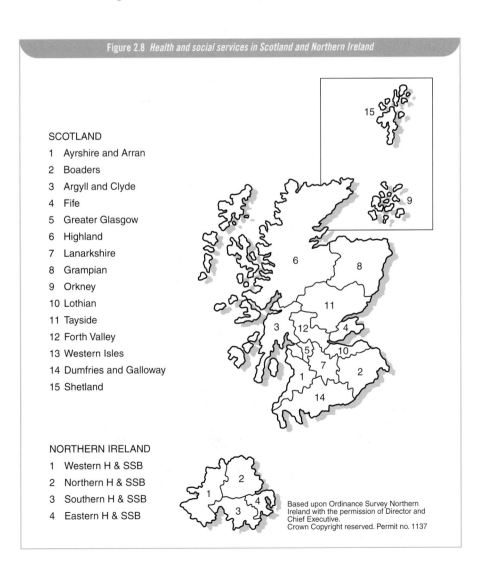

**Figure 2.8** *Health and social services in Scotland and Northern Ireland*

SCOTLAND
1   Ayrshire and Arran
2   Boaders
3   Argyll and Clyde
4   Fife
5   Greater Glasgow
6   Highland
7   Lanarkshire
8   Grampian
9   Orkney
10  Lothian
11  Tayside
12  Forth Valley
13  Western Isles
14  Dumfries and Galloway
15  Shetland

NORTHERN IRELAND
1   Western H & SSB
2   Northern H & SSB
3   Southern H & SSB
4   Eastern H & SSB

Based upon Ordinance Survey Northern Ireland with the permission of Director and Chief Executive.
Crown Copyright reserved. Permit no. 1137

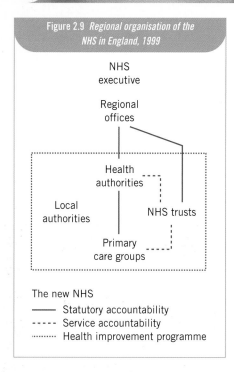

**Figure 2.9** *Regional organisation of the NHS in England, 1999*

NHS executive

Regional offices

Health authorities

Local authorities

NHS trusts

Primary care groups

The new NHS
—— Statutory accountability
----- Service accountability
·········· Health improvement programme

The Strategic Health Authorities will oversee the delivery of health services by the hospital trusts, mental health trusts and primary care trusts.

The role of Regional Health Authorities will be reduced, and the key roles of planning and delivering services will be taken over by the primary care trusts. The role of the primary care trusts will be:

▶ to assess the health needs of the population

▶ to draw up a plan to meet those needs (under the New NHS organisation this will be in the form of a **health improvement programme** (or HImP) that is developed in partnership with the local authority and the voluntary sector).

Primary care trusts will absorb community trusts, and employ staff and offer services previously provided by the community trusts. Hospital trusts and mental health trusts will still continue to operate, and these trusts will work together with the local authority to provide services for the local population. District Health Authorities will not exist. In England, there will be 29 Strategic Health Authorities instead of 95 District Health Authorities.

Wales, Scotland and Ireland will remain as they are currently organised, although this may change in the future.

## Other changes from April 2002

In 2002, patients will be able to influence the organisation of health services through the development of **patients' forums**. Complaints about services will be dealt with by the Trusts, but all Trusts will also have to have a PALS (Patient Advisory and Liaison Service) in place by April 2002.

Patients who have concerns about their treatment will be able to contact PALS who will help them. In 2001 some PALS were developed. In one London hospital the PALS office was set up in the main entrance and patients were informed about the service. It is hoped that patients' anxieties about services will be dealt with quickly, leading to fewer complaints in future.

All Trusts and health authorities have to produce annual reports, and these could give you useful information for your projects. For example, a District Health Authority Annual Report gives information about:

▶ the numbers of GPs in the area

▶ the numbers of dentists

- the numbers of opticians
- the numbers of community pharmacists.

In each year in a typical DHA there are:

- 5 million prescriptions written
- 62,000 NHS eye tests
- 78,000 immunisations and vaccinations
- 102,000 acute hospital admissions
- 9000 babies delivered.

(Source: *Merton, Sutton and Wandsworth Health Authority Annual Report 1999*)

Figure 2.10 shows the different health services available for different client groups.

## NHS Trusts

### NHS Hospital Trusts

Under the 1990 *NHS and Community Care Act*, hospitals became self-governing trusts. This meant they were able to do the following

- buy, own and sell land and services
- develop their own management systems
- employ their own staff and set out their own terms and conditions of employment (they also used outside companies for cleaning and catering services)

> **Activity**
>
> Visit your local GP surgery or health centre and find out the range of services provided.

**Primary health care** – health care that takes place in the community through the GP, district nurse, practice nurse, health visitor, CPN (community psychiatric nurse) and other members of the primary health care team (PHCT). It does not include hospital services.

**Secondary health care** – health care that takes place in hospital. This will include both medical care and surgical care, as well as investigations and day care cases.

**Medical care** means treatment by drugs, rest and therapy, which could include radiotherapy.

**Surgical care** means treatment by operations.

**Tertiary services** – health care that takes place in specialist hospitals, for example cardiac (heart) units, cancer or orthopaedic specialist hospitals.

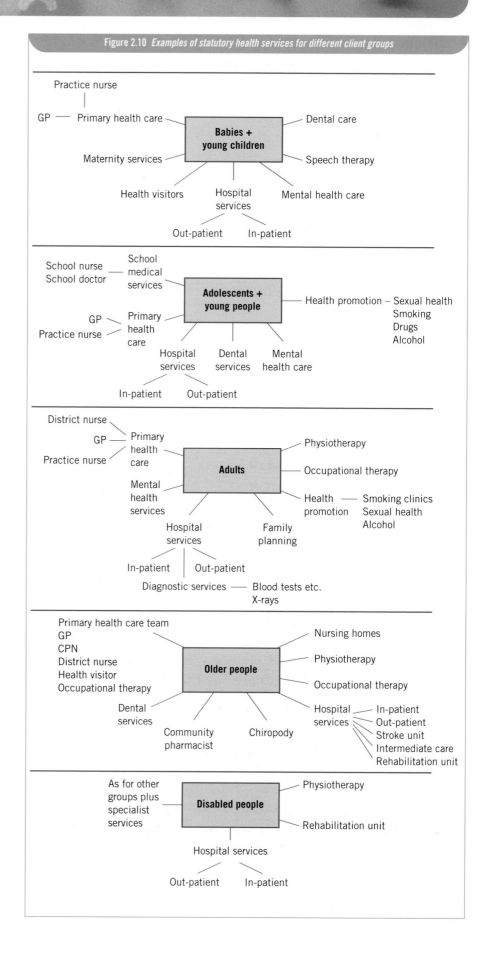

Figure 2.10 *Examples of statutory health services for different client groups*

▶ raise money through developing private patient services, renting out shops in the hospital, car park charges and other ways of raising income.

Hospital trusts have to produce an annual report, which provides statistics on numbers of patients treated, length of waiting lists, as well as planned developments.

It may be useful if you look at a copy of a hospital trust report. They should be in your local library, or else you can obtain one directly from the hospital.

## NHS Community Trusts

Community Trusts were developed in order to deliver specialist services in the community.

Figure 2.11 shows the services offered by a community trust. As you can see the following people are offered services:

▶ adults
▶ children and young people

Figure 2.11 *Services offered by a community trust*

### South West London Community Trust

**Services for Adults**

Chiropody, dental services (for people who cannot get treatment within the general dental service), distict nursing, HIV/AIDS services, sexual health and family planning, specialist nursing, speech and language therapy, stroke rehabilitation, wheelchair services.

**Services for Children and Young People**

Child protection, chiropody, continence services, dental services, early years screening, family planning, health visiting, HIV/AIDS services, immunisation and vaccination, liaison work with local authorities, school nursing, special needs services, speech and language therapy, audiology, community paediatric service.

**Services for Older People**

Continuing and short-term nursing care for clients with assessed high levels of need, respite care, community based health care, "hospital at home".

**Services for People with Learning Disabilities**

Residential care, day care, short-term health care, respite care, community services, specialist services (e.g. for clients with challenging behaviour), mental health services.

▶ older people

▶ people with learning disabilities.

After April 2002, community trusts will be absorbed into the primary care trusts, who will still continue to offer these services.

### Mental Health Trusts

Because of the specialist care needed for people with mental health problems, mental health trusts have been developed that link hospital and community care for their patients. Community psychiatric nurses are part of the outreach team that develops services such as day centres and drop-in centres for patients, as well as providing a 24-hour service in the community.

### Day surgery

Because of changes in technology, many hospitals offer day surgery for routine operations such as the removal of wisdom teeth, the removal of cataracts and other minor operations that require a general anaesthetic. More GPs are offering minor surgery in their practices. This means that the number of beds needed in hospitals for longer stay patients has gone down.

### Emergency services

NHS hospitals provide emergency services 24 hours a day. On entry to A & E (accident and emergency), you will be seen immediately by a triage nurse who will assess your need for treatment.

With the development of NHS Direct it is hoped that the use of A & E for minor problems will be reduced, and that people will either self-care, see their GP or consult a pharmacist.

In 2001 the Department of Health produced a booklet, *Your Guide to the NHS* (Figure 2.29). You should be able to find a copy in your local health centre or library.

The booklet outlines the key points in the NHS plan, which is about how the government intends to improve the NHS (the website address is given at the end of this chapter). Another leaflet also encourages people to use the NHS services effectively (Figure 2.12). Figure 2.13 shows a diagram from the leaflet showing what you can do if you feel ill.

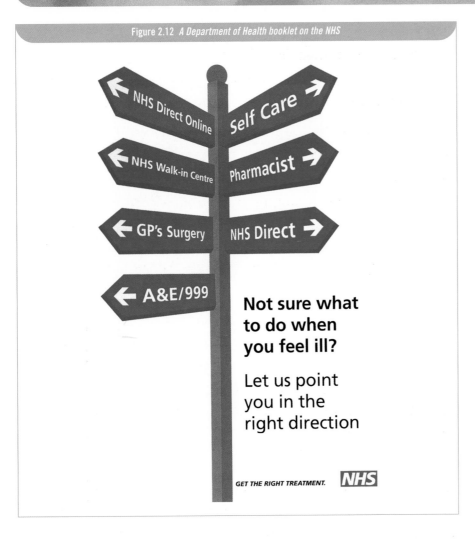

Figure 2.12 *A Department of Health booklet on the NHS*

← NHS Direct Online

Self Care →

← NHS Walk-in Centre

Pharmacist →

← GP's Surgery

NHS Direct →

← A&E/999

**Not sure what
to do when
you feel ill?**

Let us point
you in the
right direction

*GET THE RIGHT TREATMENT.* **NHS**

# Activity

Look at the following cases and decide which service
might be used.

1. You have had a rash but it seems to be getting
   better.
2. You have a sore throat.
3. Your grandmother has fallen down the stairs and is
   unconscious.
4. You (or your girlfriend) think you could be pregnant.
5. Your father has a severe pain in his chest and is
   sweating heavily.

(Answers are given on page 191.)

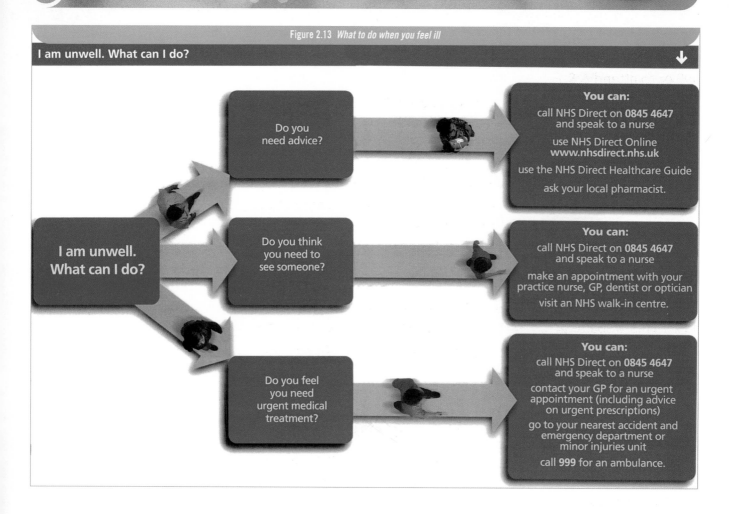

Figure 2.13 *What to do when you feel ill*

**I am unwell. What can I do?**

**I am unwell. What can I do?**

Do you need advice?

**You can:**

call NHS Direct on **0845 4647** and speak to a nurse

use NHS Direct Online **www.nhsdirect.nhs.uk**

use the NHS Direct Healthcare Guide

ask your local pharmacist.

Do you think you need to see someone?

**You can:**

call NHS Direct on **0845 4647** and speak to a nurse

make an appointment with your practice nurse, GP, dentist or optician

visit an NHS walk-in centre.

Do you feel you need urgent medical treatment?

**You can:**

call NHS Direct on **0845 4647** and speak to a nurse

contact your GP for an urgent appointment (including advice on urgent prescriptions)

go to your nearest accident and emergency department or minor injuries unit

call **999** for an ambulance.

## NHS Direct

This is a 24-hour helpline staffed by nurses who will give advice on the telephone. It covers all of Great Britain.

CASE STUDY
FIVE:
LISA

**Ectopic pregnancy**

Lisa, a 28-year-old mother of three, was suddenly gripped with abdominal pain. She was reluctant to call her GP. Assuming it was a violent stomach upset, she took some pain killers, not even realising she was pregnant. Her partner contacted NHS Direct and the nurse recognised the potential danger very quickly once he described the symptoms. Within minutes of the call, Lisa was on her way to hospital and undergoing emergency surgery for ectopic pregnancy (the embryo is in the fallopian tube instead of in the womb, and is a serious emergency).

Nurses on NHS Direct can advise callers to self-care, to see the pharmacist or to see their GP. They can also advise callers to dial 999 or to attend A & E.

The outcome of calls to the service is listed in Table 2.5. What pattern do you notice?

## NHS walk-in centres

These centres are being developed in major towns and cities. They are open from 7 am to 10 pm for advice and clinical treatment by nurses and doctors. Look at the statistics related to one walk-in centre in Figure 2.14. What are most patients advised to do?

## NHS Internet service

The website, www.nhsdirect.nhs.uk was launched in December 1999. This website gives information about the NHS and how to use it. It also includes pages on diseases and their treatment. It is an interactive website that allows users to describe their symptoms and to self-diagnose (which could cause problems!). Depending on your answers, the user will be advised to self-care, see the GP or pharmacist, or phone NHS Direct or 999.

It is hoped that all the new services will help people decide on the most appropriate type of treatment and take the burden off the A & E departments.

Pharmacists are seen as an important source of advice and, in many cases, patients are able to self-care.

**Table 2.5 Outcome of calls to NHS Direct (1999–2000)**

| England | Percentages 1999–2000 |
|---|---|
| **Nurse advice given** | |
| Gave self-care advice | 36 |
| Advised an urgent GP visit (within 24 hours) | 29 |
| Advised a routine GP visit | 12 |
| Advised a visit to accident and emergency | 9 |
| Advised patient to contact other professionals | 9 |
| Arranged for an emergency ambulance | 3 |
| Other/call aborted | 2 |
| All calls receiving nurse advice (=100%)(millions) | 1.2 |
| **Other calls (millions)** | 0.4 |
| **All calls (millions)** | 1.6 |

*Source: Social Trends 2001*, HMSO

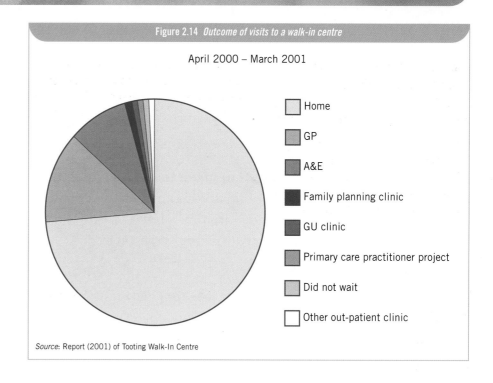

Figure 2.14 *Outcome of visits to a walk-in centre*

April 2000 – March 2001

- Home
- GP
- A&E
- Family planning clinic
- GU clinic
- Primary care practitioner project
- Did not wait
- Other out-patient clinic

*Source*: Report (2001) of Tooting Walk-In Centre

## Activity

If you have a private hospital in your area, try to visit it and find out the range of services it offers.

## Private services

### Private secondary services

Private hospitals are an alternative to NHS secondary care. Private hospitals receive most of their income from payments by patients, either directly or through private health insurance. Some private hospitals offer their own insurance schemes.

Private hospitals offer a range of services in addition to out-patient and in-patient surgical and medical care.

### Private accident and emergency care

A private alternative to NHS A & E opened in 1999 (see Figure 2.15).

Many people prefer to pay rather than wait to be seen in an NHS department, where the wait can be as long as three hours.

### Private primary care

In some areas there are still private doctors seeing patients. Other private care includes private walk-in centres which have developed in airports and railway stations. They offer treatment, advice and travel immunisation.

Figure 2.15 *Report on the opening of Britain's first private A & E at Byfleet, Surrey*

**Welcome to Britain's first private A&E, where six stitches cost £45. So would you pay to jump the queues in casualty?**

Imagine it's Saturday night and you're in your local casualty – you've hurt your finger, and you are facing a long painful wait surrounded by vomiters, drunks and bleeding children. If you knew you could nip down the road, be whisked through a pleasant (deserted) waiting area, into the arms of a calm, fully-trained doctor or nurse – at a price – would you do it? For most people, the answer to this is yes, depending on the cost. Those made of sterner principles (or with no money) might say "never". But what if it was your four-year-old daughter with the wound?

## Alternative therapists

These are private services offered in the community. Therapies include:

▶ homeopathy

▶ osteopathy

▶ chiropractic

▶ acupuncture.

# Activity

1. Use your local phone directory or *Yellow Pages* to find the types of alternative therapies that are available in your area. You can find out more about some alternative therapies on the following websites:
   www.acupuncture.org.uk.
   www.homeopathy.org.uk/page/
2. In pairs, prepare a short talk to give to the rest of the class on an alternative therapy of your choice.

## Statutory social care

The government finances a range of statutory services through the local authorities. Money is spent by the local authority on:

▶ education

▶ social services.

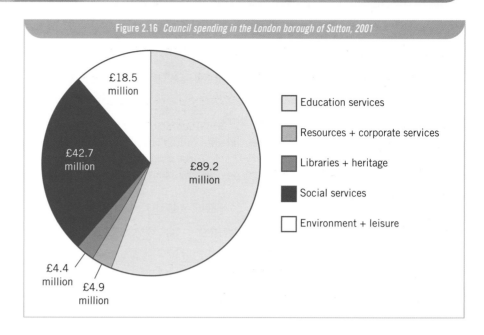

Figure 2.16  Council spending in the London borough of Sutton, 2001

- £18.5 million
- £42.7 million
- £89.2 million
- £4.4 million
- £4.9 million

- Education services
- Resources + corporate services
- Libraries + heritage
- Social services
- Environment + leisure

Figure 2.16 shows that most of the money spent by the local authority is spent on education.

The local authority receives money from central government, from payment for services and also from the rates that are paid by the local community.

Figure 2.17 shows a diagram of a typical Social Services Department.

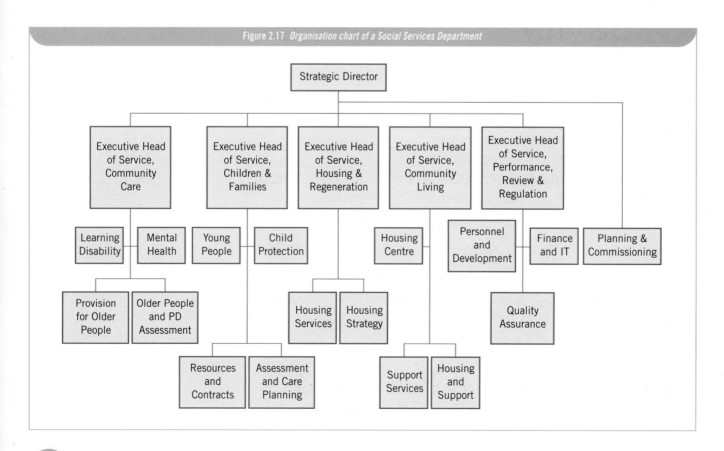

Figure 2.17  Organisation chart of a Social Services Department

There are four main areas of social care provision:

1. **residential care** – care provided in residential homes
2. **domiciliary care** – care provided in the client's own home
3. **day care** – care provided at special centres in the community
4. **field work** – care provided by social workers who care for particular client groups.

These provide service for the following groups:

▶ children and families

▶ older people

▶ people with learning difficulties

▶ people with mental health problems

▶ people with drug and alcohol problems

▶ people with AIDS and HIV

▶ refugees

▶ homeless people.

Services provided by social services include the following:

▶ assessing needs

▶ providing personal help

▶ social work

▶ day care facilities

▶ residential and respite care facilities

▶ occupational therapy

▶ rehabilitation

▶ supplying specialist equipment

▶ an emergency service, 24 hours a day, 365 days a year.

Access to social care is through referral and assessment (see Figure 2.18).

Figure 2.19 shows the services available for different client groups.

## Modernising Social Services

This government paper was published in 1998. Many people felt that social services needed review. There had been scandals involving abuse in residential homes and childrens homes, and many people did not receive the help they required when they needed it because of communication difficulties within the organisation, and between the health service and the social services.

Figure 2.18 *The assessment process carried out by social services*

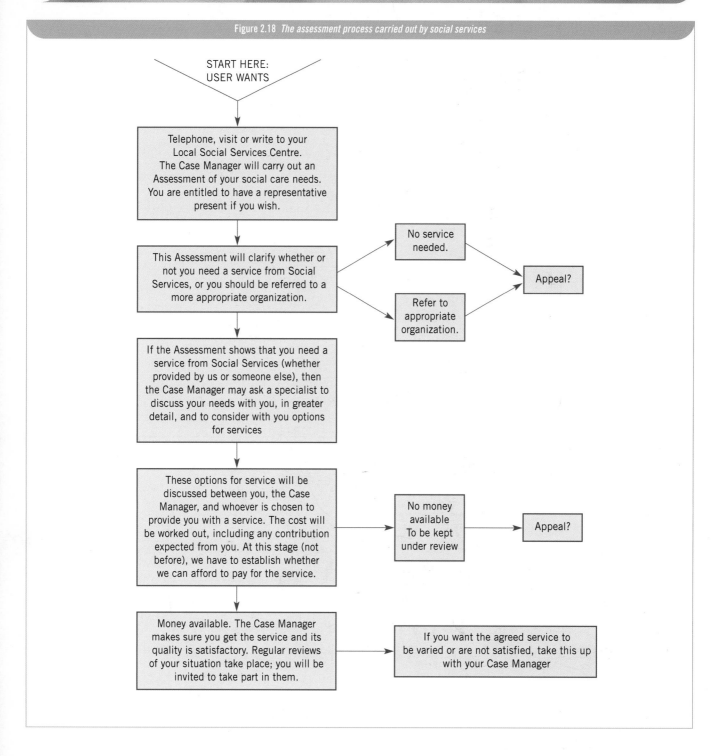

In addition, the type of social care you received was different in different parts of the country. Local authorities can decide how much they charge for services and what they should provide.

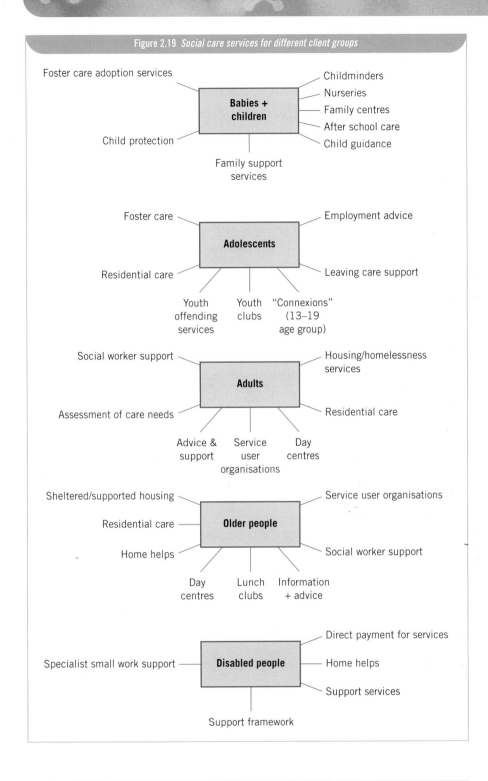

**Figure 2.19** *Social care services for different client groups*

Foster care adoption services — **Babies + children** — Childminders / Nurseries / Family centres / After school care / Child guidance

Child protection

Family support services

Foster care — **Adolescents** — Employment advice

Residential care — Leaving care support

Youth offending services | Youth clubs | "Connexions" (13–19 age group)

Social worker support — **Adults** — Housing/homelessness services

Assessment of care needs — Residential care

Advice & support | Service user organisations | Day centres

Sheltered/supported housing — **Older people** — Service user organisations

Residential care

Home helps — Social worker support

Day centres | Lunch clubs | Information + advice

Direct payment for services

Specialist small work support — **Disabled people** — Home helps

Support services

Support framework

**Duty** – this means that the local authority has to provide the service.

**Power** – this means that the local authority can offer this service if it chooses.

Examples of services that the social services have a **duty** to provide include:

▶ an initial assessment of need – this is a free service

▶ housing for people with mental health problems who have been discharged from hospital.

Examples of services that the social services may **choose** to provide include:

▶ home care facilities.

The social services provide some services directly, but nowadays they often buy these services from private or voluntary organisations.

## Private services

### Residential homes

Few residential homes are now owned and run by social services. Most residential homes are private establishments and the local council has a contract with the home to pay for the care of residents. The council will not pay for very expensive homes.

### Home care

Many private agencies do shopping and cleaning for clients. The client can either arrange for the service directly with the agency, or the local council will have a contract with the agency and charge the client for the service.

## Voluntary services

Many voluntary organisations offer a range of services. As the role of the local council has changed from providing services to buying in services, the council may buy its services from a range of organisations.

Since the 1990 *NHS and Community Care Act*, voluntary organisations have become providers of a great deal of care. Figure 2.20 shows some of the range of services that are provided by voluntary organisations in a London Borough.

(NB Although some services may be provided by volunteers, voluntary organisations also employ people to provide services.)

As part of the preparation for your project, we will now look at an example of a voluntary organisation, from the historical and national perspective. You could then investigate a voluntary organisation in your local area.

Figure 2.20 *Examples of voluntary services for different client groups*

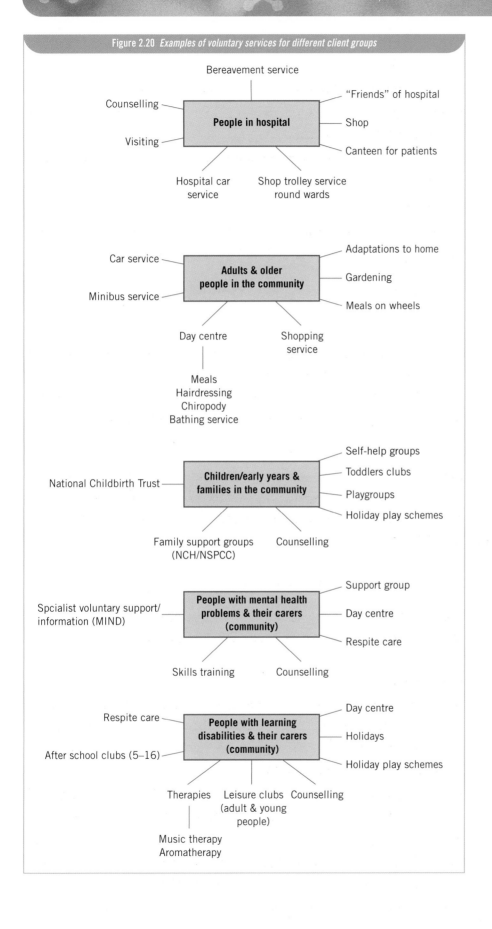

CASE STUDY
SIX:
MENCAP

**A national voluntary organisation – Mencap**

In November 1946, a young mother with a mentally handicapped child wrote to the *Nursery World* magazine about her problems. Another young mother, Judy Fryd, responded through the column of the magazine and, as a result, many mothers contacted the magazine and the Association of Backward Children was founded.

Members of the group received newsletters and advice, and regional groups were set up throughout the UK. By 1955 there were 167 local groups and the name of the organisation was changed to the National Society for Mentally Handicapped Children. In 1960, World Mental Health Year was celebrated and the *Mental Health Act* of 1960 abolished the terms mental defective, idiots, imbeciles and feeble minded. In the 1970s many of the large institutions for people with a mental handicap were closed and the patients were discharged into the community without adequate support. In 1980 the Society changed its name again to **The National Society for Mentally Handicapped Children and Adults** (or **Mencap**).

With more people of all ages with mental handicap coming into the community, Mencap developed a range of services (see Figure 2.21). As well as providing services for people with mental handicap (or learning disabilities, as it is now called) Mencap is an action group, trying to influence government policy and to give information to the general public so that prejudice against people with learning difficulties is reduced. Mencap manages more than 600 homes where adults can live with support. It also provides flats and other accommodation with 24-hour support for the residents. It has a National College, which provides training in life, social and practical skills for people aged 16 to 25, and other educational projects. It provides an employment service supporting people as they go into work. It has set up a national system of **Gateway** clubs that provide leisure activities. It offers respite care, counselling, advice and information for families.

(*Source: Our Concern, The Story of the National Society for Mentally Handicapped Children and Adults*, 1946–1980)

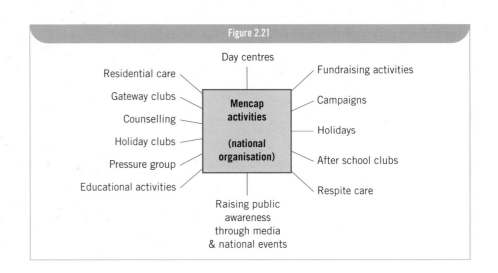

Figure 2.21

**Learning disability** can be defined as a life-long condition which results from damage to the brain before, during or after birth or from genetic or chromosome factors (e.g. Down's Syndrome).

Many voluntary organisations started off as small local groups and then became national organisations. Volunteers are essential if local groups are going to be able to succeed.

## Activity

A useful book called *The Charities Digest* (published by Waterlow) gives details of national and local charities in the UK. It is available in most libraries. Try to obtain a copy and look at the range of charities in health and social care that are listed. Using your local library find out what local groups you have in your area, what group of people they help, and how they are organised.

## CASE STUDY SEVEN:

The **Weekend Break Project** is a local voluntary group that was set up to give the carers of people with Alzheimer's Disease or dementia a break on Saturdays and Sundays, and also to provide an enjoyable experience for the clients. As the manager of the group said, "Having Alzheimers doesn't mean you can't enjoy yourself!"

It was started in 1991 when the editor of a local paper had a friend who was diagnosed as having Alzheimer's Disease, and he saw the effect the disease had on all the family. Through the paper, he launched an appeal that raised £30,000 to open day care provision at a local hospital unit. The project was supported by the local centre for voluntary services and the local authority, and two centres are now involved in the project on Saturdays and Sundays. The centres are managed by qualified staff, supported by co-ordinators and volunteers. Volunteers act as drivers, escorts and general helpers.

Funding is provided by the local council, from donations and from fund-raising events.

The ages of volunteers range from 16 to 75, and they are given basic training when they start. Activities include local outings, as well as parties and entertainment. The centres are open from

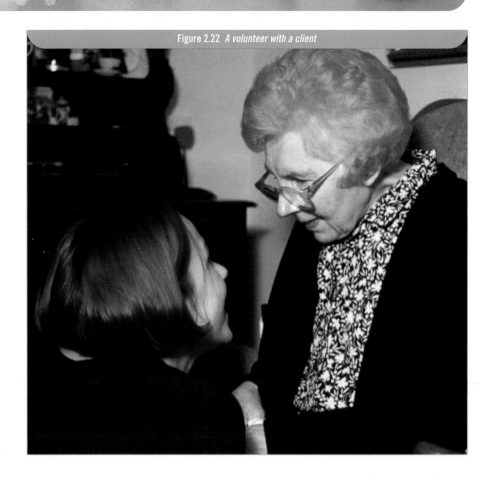

Figure 2.22 *A volunteer with a client*

9 am to 4 pm and meals are provided. Clients are referred to the project through the CPN, the care manager or the consultant psychiatrist. Most of the clients live in their own homes or with a carer. They really enjoy their time at the Centre. None of this work would be possible without the volunteers.

Christine is a volunteer with the Project group. She is 17 and studying for her A levels. She wants to be a doctor and she has applied to medical school. She comes every Saturday. She helps with meal times, and plays games with the clients. She goes on outings with the group to help out. She joined the group because she wanted to find out more about Alzheimer's. In Figure 2.22 Christine is talking to one of the clients.

Stimulation of the person with Alzheimer's is very important, and this is done through conversation, games, art work, and reminiscence therapy.

Ashna (18) is another volunteer. She is also hoping to be a doctor. She comes each week, and her main interest is in art and craft work that she does with the group. Because the clients need careful supervision, there is one helper for every four or five people.

# Early years services

There is an overlap in services provided for the health care, social care and education services provided for children.

## Primary health care

Most of the care of young children is undertaken by parents. With less time spent in hospital, children are more likely to be looked after in their own homes. GPs have responsibility for all the children in their practice. Preventative services such as routine immunisations, developmental checks and advising parents are all part of the work of the Primary Health Care Team (PHCT).

Table 2.6 is an immunisation table that shows the times at which children will have their jabs. Protection against Meningitis C is also currently available.

| DISEASE | TIME | COMMON REACTIONS | PROTECTION |
|---------|------|------------------|------------|
| Diphtheria, whooping cough (Pertussis), tetanus (also known as DTP or triple vaccine) | Injections at 2, 3, and 4 months; repeat diphtheria + tetanus at $3\frac{1}{2}$–5 years | Child may become feverish; the site of the injection may be sore | Repeat at school leaving age |
| Polio | Oral vaccine at 2, 3 and 4 months; repeat at $3\frac{1}{2}$–5 years | None | Repeat at school leaving age and every 10 years, if travelling to high risk countries |
| MMR – measles, mumps, German measles (rubella) | Injection at 12–15 months; repeated at $3\frac{1}{2}$–5 years or earlier | Child may become feverish and have a slight rash for 7–10 days after vaccination | Further doses are not recommended after 2 injections |
| Tuberculosis (BCG) | Injection at 10–13 years to all school children not immune | The site of the injection may be sore and stiff | Unknown |
| Hib (Haemophilus influenza Hib type B) Hib meningitis, epiglottis, septicaemia, septic arthritis, osteomyelitis, pneumonia | Injection at 2, 3 and 4 months, or just one injection for children over a year old | The site of the injection may become red and swollen | After 4 years of age the child should have developed a natural resistance to Hib and does not need to be immunised |
| Meningoccal C, meningitis, septicaemia | As Hib above | As Hib above | Long lasting. A booster not currently recommended |

Table 2.6 *Health authority immunisation table*

## School services

The government's **Healthier Schools Programme** means healthier children. School nurses promote the health of the children and give help and advice to parents and pupils.

Each school has a named doctor and nurse who visit the school regularly and refer children to other services in the community.

| JOB/TITLE | SERVICES & SUPPORT FOR: | REFERRAL BY |
|---|---|---|
| Health vistor | Infant feeding and nutrition, Child development, behavioural problems | GP, midwife, self-referral |
| Audiology service | Children who have hearing problems or are behind with language development | Health visitor, school nurse, GP, self-referral |
| Speech and language therapist | Children who stammer, children under 6 who cannot pronounce words properly, young babies and children who have difficulty eating and drinking | GP, health visitor, school nurse |
| Community paediatrician | Minor and major health problems in babies and young children, children with special needs, developmental problems | GP, health visitor, school nurse |
| Child and adolescent psychiatrist or family therapist | Depression, eating disorders, disruptive behaviour, bereavement problems, abuse, self abuse | GP, health visitor, school nurse, teacher |
| Educational and clinical psychologist | Family crisis, bullying, anxiety, problems at school | Educational authority, school nurse, teacher |
| Sleep and behaviour clinics (run by health visitor or/and psychiatrist) | Sleep problems, toddler tantrums, toileting problems, aggression | GP, health visitor, school nurse |
| Community dental service (dentist) | Pre-school or school child with special needs who needs dental care at home | Dentist, GP |
| Enuresis clinic (bedwetting service) (run by health visitor) | Bedwetting in children and teenagers | School nurse, health visitor, GP |

*Table 2.7 The paediatric community team*

# Activity

Table 2.7 shows the children's services available in the community. After you have studied it, look at the following case studies and decide which service should be used for each child (you can refer to more than one service if you think it is necessary).

1.  Jason, aged three, is very jealous of his baby sister. He keeps biting and pinching her. He is also very aggressive in the nursery classroom.
2.  Bella, aged four, has cerebral palsy and has difficulty swallowing.
3.  Shakira is six and still wets the bed at night. She finds it embarrassing as she wants to stay overnight at her friend's house.
4.  David, aged six, has learning disabilities. It is impossible for his mother to take him to the dentist in the high street. She has noticed that his teeth are stained and dirty, and she has difficulty teaching David how to clean his teeth.
5.  Jane has just had twins. She is trying to breast feed them without success.
6.  Leroy, who is four, has had continuous ear infections for the last year, and ignores his mother when she calls him in from the garden.
7.  Anna is 14 months old and cannot sit up on her own yet. She seems to have problems seeing things. Her mother thinks she has a squint.
8.  Maria is eight and wants to be a model when she grows up. Her mother has discovered that she has not been eating her packed lunch at school. When she changes for games the teacher notices she has scratches and cuts on her arms.
9.  Rania is seven. Her parents divorced recently and she is living with her mother. She is very disruptive in class. She will not sit down, but runs round the classroom, shouting and causing a disturbance.

(Answers given on page 191.)

There are also paediatric nurses employed by the hospital or community trusts, who visit children in their own homes to continue treatment or to offer support after a stay in hospital. The duties of a community paediatric nurse can include the following:

▶ follow-up care after treatment in A & E

▶ post-operative care

▶ removal of stitches, dressing of wounds, giving injections

▶ advising and training parents in giving care.

*Emergency health services for children*

Apart from the out-of-hours service offered by GPs, there are specialist children's hospitals that look after children until the age of 16. The hospitals are organised so that children feel comfortable. Often the departments and wards are brightly painted with pictures and other decorations.

## Secondary health services for early years

Secondary care is provided in hospitals. Hospital paediatricians provide emergency and routine surgery for children. GPs will refer children to outpatient departments where they can be seen by the specialist team. Nowadays parents are encouraged to stay with their children in hospital, and overnight accommodation is offered to them.

### Hospital play specialist

A hospital play specialist is usually a trained nursery nurse who has additional training in supporting children through play. Operations and procedures can be explained to the child using dolls. Play is also used to relieve stress.

## Social services early years

The local social service departments provide a range of services for young children. These services may be provided directly by social services, or they are provided in partnership with voluntary organisations, or they are purchased from private or other independent sector providers.

### Statutory provision

The *Children Act* (1989) was an important piece of legislation that stated *the services that must be provided for those children assessed as being in need*:

▶ day care for children under five and not at school
▶ care and supervised activities outside school hours and during school holidays
▶ accommodation if required, if children are lost, abandoned or without a carer that can provide accommodation.

Social Services must also provide:

▶ assessment of needs
▶ an emergency service 24 hours a day, 365 days a year.

Social services may also provide the following caring services for children and their families:

▶ occupational therapy
▶ supplying specialist equipment
▶ respite care
▶ personal help.

### Day care services and childminders

Childminders must be registered with the local authority, and they are inspected and registered annually. Procedures for this will be changing in 2002, when inspections will be carried out either by OFSTED or by the Care Standards Council.

### Fostering and adoption

The *Children Act* (1989) states that the local authority must make arrangements to enable the child to live with their family unless this would harm the child. Foster carers are approved by either the local authority or by a voluntary or private organisation. Local authorities have to keep a register of foster carers in the area and keep records of children placed with them.

The law related to adoption is complicated (*Adoption Act* 1979 and *Children Act* 1989). An adoption order transfers all the responsibilities of the parent to the adopters. An adopter has to be:

▶ at least 21

▶ resident in the UK

▶ able to meet the criteria of the relevant adoption agency or local authority.

### Residential care for early years

At the moment the inspection unit of the local authority inspects residential homes twice a year. One of these visits is announced, which means that the home has notice when to expect a visit. The other visit is unannounced, when the home does not receive notice and the inspector arrives unexpectedly.

There has been a great deal of concern about the level of abuse in children's homes, so the inspection procedures are being reviewed. As well as trained full-time inspectors, lay people who have been trained as **lay assessors** will accompany the inspectors on their visits.

In the future the inspection unit will become separate from the local authority.

### Non-statutory provision

Local authorities provide some non-statutory provision, such as training for childminders. Other examples of non-statutory provision would include:

▶ private nurseries

▶ private residential homes

▶ private fostering and adoption agencies.

These are privately run as a business, but the services are used and paid for by the social services.

**Independent voluntary provision** for early years can include:

▶ toddlers' clubs

▶ care for children with special needs (Mencap services)

▶ holiday care

▶ mother and child support groups.

Figure 2.23 is an example of a voluntary service for families with young children.

Family Focus is a registered charity that was set up to protect and preserve the mental and physical health of families with children under the age of five.

**Family Focus** aims to:

▶ work alongside parents to develop family life skills

▶ help parents enjoy parenthood

▶ help parents cope with the daily pressures of life.

To do this, parents can take part in a parenting skills course that includes:

**Figure 2.23 *Example of a voluntary service for children and their families***

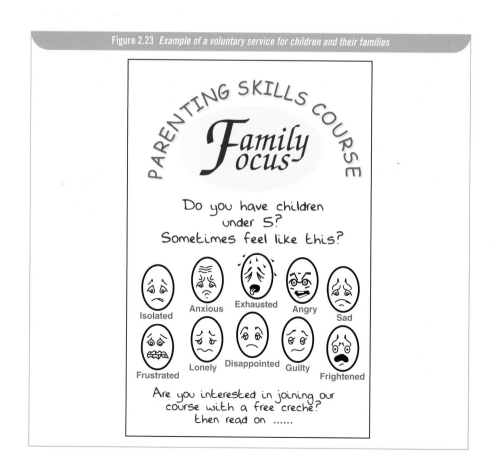

- child development
- managing behaviour
- meeting needs of children and parents
- the importance of play.

There are also charities involved with the protection of young children. The most well known of these is the **NSPCC** (National Society for the Prevention of Cruelty to Children). The NSPCC advises parents on child care, supports families who are finding it difficult to cope with their children, as well as investigating cases of abuse and cruelty to children.

*Informal provision*

Much of the care of young children is arranged on an informal basis. For example, friends and neighbours may do unpaid babysitting; local churches may run mother and toddler clubs.

## Informal care for all client groups

Figure 2.24 shows how the focus for care has moved away from long-stay hospitals into the community. Although the Primary Health Care Team offers health care in the community, family, friends and neighbours offer more and more informal care. Under the 1990 *NHS Community Care Act*, long-stay hospitals were closed and patients moved into the community. People with learning disabilities, physical disabilities and mental health problems are now cared for in the community, and in practice this means by the family.

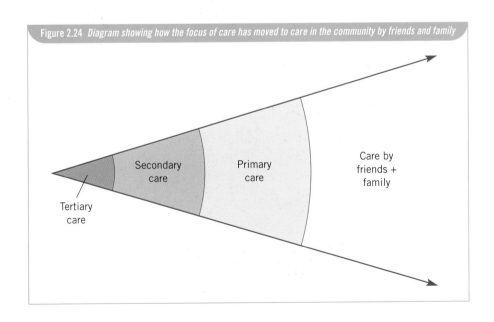

Figure 2.24 *Diagram showing how the focus of care has moved to care in the community by friends and family*

## Carers

There are six million carers in the UK, but **who are they**?

A carer is anyone who is helping to look after a partner, friend or relative who, because of illness, old age or disability may not be able to manage at home without help.

# Activity

These are examples of people who are cared for in their own homes. For each example, think of who is most likely to care for them:

1. a widow of 88 living in her own home
2. a young man with multiple sclerosis
3. a child of five with learning disabilities
4. a married man of 30 who has had a car accident
5. a single woman of 30 recovering from a serious operation
6. a man of 75 living with his wife.

These examples show some of the different people that carers look after.

Your answers may reflect your views of the role and responsibilities of families, neighbours and friends.

Carers save the government an estimated £34 billion every year by caring for people at home. Without this informal care, many people would have to live in residential care.

It has been estimated that there are 900,000 people who care for someone for more than 50 hours each week.

We will now look at some research carried out by the Princess Royal Trust in a report called *8 Hours a Day and Taken for Granted* published in 1998.

This report summarises the findings of 7000 questionnaires that were sent to carers' centres in the UK, and focuses on the responses of 1346 carers who care for someone for eight hours or more each day.

Sixty-three per cent of these had been caring for more than five years.

Ninety-four per cent are providing medical care, but only 33% of these had received any training or guidance of any kind.

If we look at Figure 2.25, which shows that the relationship of the carer to the cared for, we can see that family relationships are important when caring for people.

Many people think that it is mainly older people that are cared for in the community, but research shows that there is a wide range of age groups receiving informal care.

In the past, women did most of the caring in the home for sick and disabled members of the family.

Factors that could have brought about change include:

▶ families may not live near each other so that husband and wife support each other more

▶ ideas have changed about what is women's work and what is men's work

## Activity

Look at Figure 2.25 again and answer these questions:
1. Which group is most likely to care for someone?
2. Which group is least likely to care for someone?
(Answers given on page 191.)

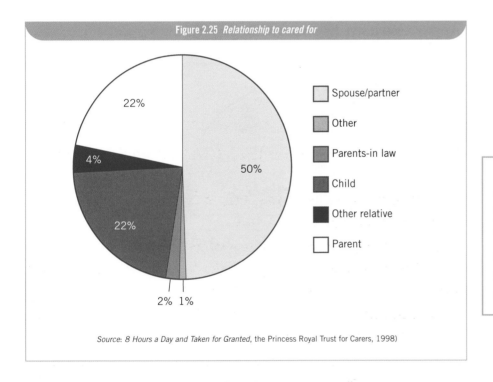

**Figure 2.25 Relationship to cared for**

- Spouse/partner — 50%
- Other — 22%
- Parents-in law
- Child — 22%
- Other relative — 4%
- Parent

2% 1%

Source: *8 Hours a Day and Taken for Granted*, the Princess Royal Trust for Carers, 1998)

## Activity

Look at Table 2.8. Are women still the main carers? Why do you think more men are becoming carers now?

**Table 2.8 Percentage of adults who were carers by age and gender**

| Great Britain | Males | Females | Percentages All |
|---|---|---|---|
| 16–29 | 5 | 6 | 6 |
| 30–44 | 8 | 13 | 10 |
| 45–64 | 17 | 22 | 20 |
| 65 and over | 14 | 11 | 13 |
| All aged 16 and over | 11 | 14 | 13 |

Source: *Social Trends 2000*, HMSO

▶ there are increased numbers of young carers, including boys under 16.

# Activity

What age do you think a typical carer is? Over 65? Over 40? If you look at Figure 2.26 you can see that many carers are under 65.

1. What percentage are 16 to 45?
2. What percentage are 16 to 64?
3. How does this compare with the percentage over 65?

(Answers given on page 191.)

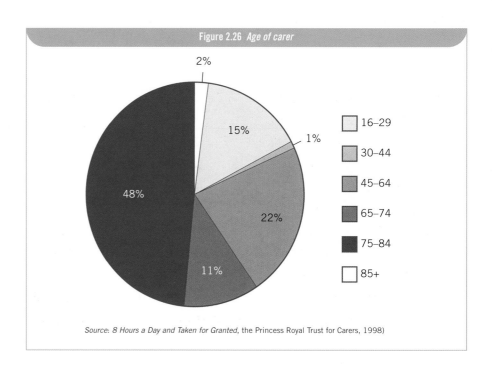

**Figure 2.26** *Age of carer*

2%
15%
1%
48%
22%
11%

16–29
30–44
45–64
65–74
75–84
85+

*Source: 8 Hours a Day and Taken for Granted, the Princess Royal Trust for Carers, 1998)*

As we can see, a large percentage of carers are between 16 and 64. This means that the caring they do could affects the amount of time they have to spend on education and work. If you are caring for someone at home, how might this affect your work? If you are unable to work because of your caring role, what effects may this have?

Many people who are carers find that caring is very tiring, and this affects the work they do. They become stressed and may have to move from full-time work to part-time work, or give up work altogether. What extra strain could this put on the carer? The effects might include:

- low income
- no leisure time
- no break from caring.

**Caring can be very time consuming**. The Princess Royal Trust research found that 58% of carers aged 16 + spend more than 15 hours caring. If there are only 24 hours in a day, this doesn't leave much time for doing other things.

## What does caring involve?

Caring could be:

- helping someone get up in the morning and go to bed at night
- cooking a meal and helping the person eat it
- helping someone have a bath and use the toilet.

Look at Figure 2.27. You can see that seven areas of care are identified here.

## Young carers

So far we have looked at carers over 16, but recent research shows that there may be many young carers **under** 16. What do you think is the age of the youngest carer: 14, 12, 10, 8, 6? The youngest carer known to a carers' centre was six.

In a recent study *Too much to take on* (1999), 20 young carers' groups were questioned about caring and bullying. 240 questionnaires were completed: 44% of young carers who responded were aged 11 to 13. This can be a difficult time for young carers as they are changing schools and making new friends.

Thirty-five per cent of young carers were 10 or under, and this means they are taking on a lot of responsibility at a very young age.

### *Gender*

More young carers are female. This reflects the older male/female carer split.

### *Primary carer*

This is the **only person** providing care, and puts a great deal of pressure on a young person.

Sixteen per cent of young carers in the survey were the primary carer. Of those 16 %, 28% were 10 years old or less.

Young carers who are primary carers are more likely to care for someone with a physical disability (32%) or a mental health problem (21%).

> ## Activity
> Go through each pie chart and identify the patterns that you see. Which type of help is provided regularly and which type of help is less likely to be provided? Can you think of possible reasons behind the differences?

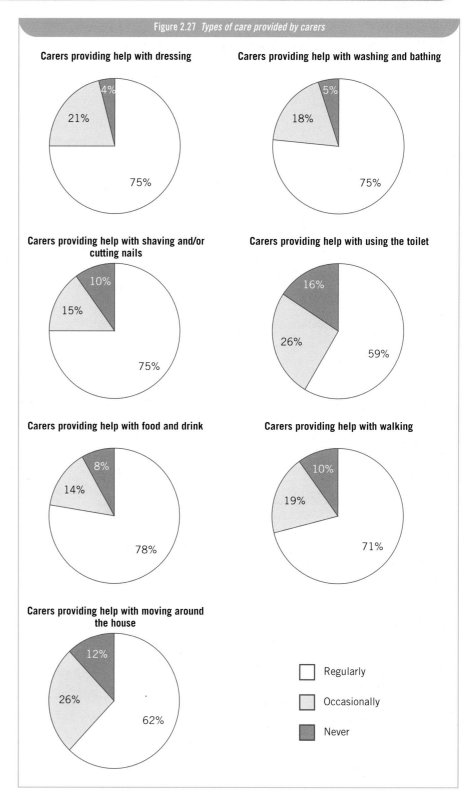

Figure 2.27 *Types of care provided by carers*

Carers providing help with dressing

4%
21%
75%

Carers providing help with washing and bathing

5%
18%
75%

Carers providing help with shaving and/or cutting nails

10%
15%
75%

Carers providing help with using the toilet

16%
26%
59%

Carers providing help with food and drink

8%
14%
78%

Carers providing help with walking

10%
19%
71%

Carers providing help with moving around the house

12%
26%
62%

☐ Regularly
☐ Occasionally
☐ Never

## Support for young carers

Thirty-three per cent of the young carers interviewed said that their teachers did not know they were looking after someone. Many young carers do not tell their friends that they are carers as they feel they would be laughed at and no-one would want to be friends with them. They try to keep their caring role a secret.

## CASE STUDY EIGHT: CHRISTOPHER

**Christopher's story**

Christopher is 13 years old and lives with his mother. He has been a carer as long as he can remember. He looks after his mother, who needs continuous care as she has multiple health problems, including epilepsy. Although home carers visit to help with his mother's personal care, they are not there all the time. Christopher helps with the household chores and cooking. His mother gets lonely during the day, so he does not like to leave her alone after school, and at weekends he helps her with personal care and toileting, although he still feels awkward doing these tasks. His mother has regular epileptic fits which can be quite frightening. Christopher often has to dial 999 and get an ambulance to take his mother to A & E. Each time they have to wait several hours.

Christopher finds he is getting behind with school work. He is always tired because of his caring role and he is always 'on call', so it is difficult to relax, watch TV or read a book. He feels the odd one out at school. He has few friends as he finds it difficult to bring them home. He feels embarrassed when school friends see him pushing his mother in a wheelchair. He cannot stay behind at school to play football because he worries about his mother. He has been bullied verbally by boys calling him names. Sometimes he feels very depressed and frustrated.

## Activity

Read Christopher's story.

1. What needs does he have and how could these be met?
2. Here is a list of Christopher's problems:
   ▶ bullying at school
   ▶ falling behind with school work
   ▶ feeling tired all the time
   ▶ coping with the idea his mother is going to die
   ▶ no time for hobbies and leisure activities
   ▶ dealing with epileptic fits
   ▶ lack of friends and support
   ▶ bullying

Can you think of possible solutions?

Research shows that 79% of young female carers have been bullied at school, and that 60% of young male carers have experienced bullying. These young people suffered verbal, physical and emotional abuse, and many truanted from school as a result.

Many schools have an anti-bullying policy. What else could be done to help people like Christopher?

▶ Young carers should be identified and assessed for their needs. Only 11% of young carers have been assessed.

▶ Teachers should be aware of children who are carers and provide additional support.

▶ Young carers projects are run at carers' centres and provide activities including painting and outings, as well as counselling, support and advice.

## Activity

Is there a carers' centre near you? If there is, find out what services it offers.
Figure 2.28 shows the services offered by a centre in South London.

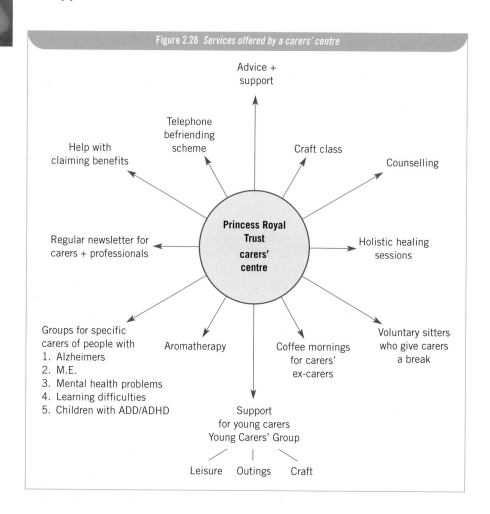

**Figure 2.28** *Services offered by a carers' centre*

- Advice + support
- Telephone befriending scheme
- Craft class
- Counselling
- Help with claiming benefits
- Holistic healing sessions
- Regular newsletter for carers + professionals
- **Princess Royal Trust carers' centre**
- Groups for specific carers of people with
  1. Alzheimers
  2. M.E.
  3. Mental health problems
  4. Learning difficulties
  5. Children with ADD/ADHD
- Aromatherapy
- Coffee mornings for carers' ex-carers
- Voluntary sitters who give carers a break
- Support for young carers Young Carers' Group
  - Leisure
  - Outings
  - Craft

In this section we have seen how a range of providers offer services to different clients.

## CASE STUDY NINE: MRS BROWN

Mrs Brown is 80 years old and lives on her own. She sees the doctor once a month to check her blood pressure and her diabetes. The district nurse comes to check her blood levels and her insulin (Mrs Brown has learnt to inject herself each day).

On Tuesdays Mrs Brown arranges to go to the post office to collect her pension. She phones and arranges to be collected by the local Dial a Ride service. On Thursdays the home help comes to give the place a clean up. Every fortnight a volunteer from the local Age Concern comes to do her shopping. Every six weeks Mrs Brown goes to the local day centre, where the chiropodist attends to her feet, and she has her hair done by the visiting hairdresser. If she needs a prescription the pharmacist delivers it to her.

Last year Mrs Brown had a fall, and had to go into hospital for a few days. Before she left, the occupational therapist checked her home and recommended that some rails should be put up in the hall. These were put up by a volunteer from Age Concern. Mrs Brown started having Meals on Wheels when she came home, but she never knew when her lunch was going to arrive, so now she uses a company who delivers a range of frozen meals for the month, and she can heat them up herself.

Mrs Brown wears an alarm round her neck, so if she has a fall she can summon help. She has become rather deaf recently and she has a new hearing aid from the hospital.

## Activity

Look at the following case study and identify the different service providers who work together to support Mrs Brown. Decide whether they are health or social care, statutory, voluntary or private.

Did you manage to identify all the service providers and decide whether they were health or social care, statutory, voluntary or private?

You could make up your own case studies of clients from the different groups – babies and children, adolescents, adults and disabled people, and decide what services they might use and who would provide them.

# WAYS OF OBTAINING CARE SERVICES, AND BARRIERS TO ACCESS

How can people gain access to care services and what can prevent people from being able to use services they need?

## Methods of referral

The ways that people gain access to care services are known as **methods of referral**. You should know about the different methods that exist.

### Self-referral

This is when people decide to go and ask for the services themselves. Examples of self-referral are:

▶ going to the local Accident and Emergency department when you have an accident

▶ making an appointment to see the GP (general practitioner)

▶ going to a genito-urinary medical (GUM) clinic for treatment of sexually transmitted diseases

▶ contacting the health visitor or practice nurse for advice or an appointment.

Self-referral is developing as the health and care services change. In the NHS, walk-in centres have been developed where people can go for advice and treatment. The use of the phone service NHS Direct is another example.

Many of the new services on offer are a way of encouraging people to self-refer to appropriate services. Accident and Emergency services often find they are caring for people who could use other services, including the pharmacist. This could mean that serious emergencies may not be treated as rapidly as they should.

Apart from the leaflet *Get the Right Treatment*, which we have already discussed, there are other leaflets. Figure 2.29 suggests how patients can refer themselves to the right service. All GP surgeries are required to produce a booklet giving information to patients about how to treat common conditions. See if you can find this at your local surgery.

**Figure 2.29** *How patients can refer themselves to the right service*

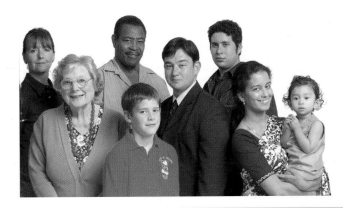

Getting the most from your National Health Service

Your guide
**to the NHS** →

## Professional referral

This means that the person will be referred by the doctor, nurse, teacher or social worker to see a specialist or other professional. Examples of this would include:

▶ the GP making an appointment for a patient to see a consultant in the out-patient department of a hospital

▶ the psychiatrist referring a patient to a CPN (community psychiatric nurse)

▶ a teacher referring a disruptive pupil to the educational psychologist

▶ a health visitor referring a patient to the social work team.

Referrals to hospital for appointments can take a long time, and there are various government initiatives to reduce waiting lists for out-patient appointments. These include:

▶ encouraging the use of specialist GPs who will undertake procedures usually done in hospital

- using outreach clinics, where the consultant visits a local health centre and sees patients near their own home
- changing arrangements for making appointments so that patients can choose a date and time convenient for them.

One of the key problems facing the NHS is how to reduce the number of patients who do not attend appointments (DNA). The level of DNAs is being monitored in GP practices and in hospital clinics.

Can you think of ways to encourage people to attend or to cancel unwanted appointments? It has been suggested that people who do not attend should have to pay a cancellation fee. What do you think of this idea?

## Third-party referral

There are a number of examples of third-party referral, which is when a person is put in contact with a service by a friend or neighbour. Voluntary services are often accessed through word of mouth.

## Activity

In your groups, you could develop a leaflet or information pack giving information about services available in your area for the following client groups:
- parents of young children
- older people
- people with physical disabilities
- people with mental health problems

### CASE STUDY TEN: SHEILA

Sheila was looking after her husband, Tony, who had dementia. She was finding it difficult to cope. Sheila did not know how to access services to help her. A neighbour, who had cared for her own husband, suggested that she should contact the carers' centre for advice. The manager of the carers' centre was able to help Sheila apply for additional financial benefits, and was able to tell her about the services she could use, including respite care.

There are various voluntary groups that give advice about services. Many people do not use services that are available because they are not aware of their existence.

In some areas there are information packs giving information about services available. These are often placed in libraries or health centres. Sometimes the people who need the information do not attend these places. Can you think of other ways to inform people of services? Not everyone has the Internet, and we will see in the next section that there are all kinds of barriers to accessing care services.

# Barriers to services

## Physical barriers

Many older GP practices have stairs, either to the front door or to the consulting rooms, which can make it difficult for people who have mobility problems, or for mothers using prams and pushchairs.

People with sensory problems may also have difficulties of access. Phoning up to make an appointment can be a problem if you are deaf. Finding your way round a hospital can be difficult if you are visually impaired.

## Psychological barriers

Men are less likely to make appointments to see the doctor because they feel it is 'unmanly'. As a result, many male patients finally see a doctor when the problem has become serious. Men are less likely than women to see their doctor if they are suffering from depression. Young men feel embarrassed seeing the doctor, especially about problems related to their genitals. This is a particular concern as there has been an increase in testicular cancer among young men. How might they be encouraged to see the doctor? There have been health programmes in secondary schools about testicular cancer and encouraging young men to examine themselves, but the results have been disappointing.

Other psychological barriers can be phobias, when people develop an intense fear of, for example, needles (so they don't have injections) or of dental treatment.

Some phobias can be successfully treated, but the key to overcoming many of these barriers is through effective communication with patients, so that they understand why certain services may help them.

Some older people do not want strangers coming into their homes to look after them, or do not want to lose their independence.

## Financial barriers

When the health service was set up in 1948, health care was to be free at the point of delivery. This included eye tests, prescriptions for medicines and dental treatment to certain groups. In 2002, many people are unwilling to use some of the services because of the cost involved. At the moment a prescription costs £6.10 per item, although some groups are exempt.

> # Activity
> Visit your local health centre and find out what facilities are available to reduce problems of access.

## Activity

Find the booklet HC11 *Help with Health Costs*. This itemises the help people can receive towards health costs. In many instances the person has to fill in numerous lengthy forms in order to receive financial help. Details of help are also available on the web at www.doh.gov.uk/nhscharges/hc11.htm

Many social care services are now means tested and many people (especially older people) do not want to give information of a personal nature to the social worker. Depending upon the level of income and savings, older people have to contribute towards the costs of care, either in their own home or in residential care. This means that many older people do not receive the services they need, although their income and level of savings may mean that they would contribute little, if anything, towards their care. The financial assessment covers many pages of form filling, which can be difficult to do.

Another aspect of financial barriers to access, relates to dental treatment and eye tests. With certain exceptions, these have to be paid for in full, or else a contribution made towards the cost. Health workers fear that because of these charges, dental health will decline and serious eye conditions may not be detected.

Refugees and asylum seekers are another group that experience problems of access to services for financial reasons.

### Geographical barriers

As we have seen, the areas in Britain are very varied, with some densely populated towns and cities, and some rural areas that have limited facilities.

In some rural areas local bus and train services have been reduced and there are problems for specialists reaching outlying areas, as well as for patients accessing services. With the changes in the NHS, which mean that in the future there will be a concentration of specialist services in a few areas, this problem is likely to increase (see Case Study 11).

How might these concerns be addressed?

Help with travelling costs can be obtained through the Benefits Agency, but again the process is time consuming. What provision might the hospital be able to offer? Again, we have to remember that all hospital trusts have to keep to a tight budget, so if money is spent on one area this reduces the money available for other services.

### Cultural and language barriers

In a study conducted in one London borough, it was found that the greatest problem facing refugees and asylum seekers was the lack of adequate interpreting services.

## CASE STUDY ELEVEN:

### Access to specialist services

Renal transplant surgery (kidney transplants) is a specialism. Consultants have to perform a certain number of operations each year in order to be regarded as having the necessary skills. This has meant that instead of two hospitals in South London performing renal transplants, only one will do this in future. Relatives and patients have expressed concern about the following:

▶ travelling time and costs for visitors and patients when surgery is done
▶ overnight accommodation for relatives
▶ follow up visits and treatment at the one centre will again be a problem.

Some telephone interpreting services have been set up in GP practices which have been helpful, but in many cases the use of a face to face interpreter is needed, especially when dealing with a complicated situation or when a family is involved in the discussion.

Receptionists in GP practices have found problems in identifying the language required. One way to solve this is through the use of a leaflet in which many languages are identified. Once the patient points to their language, the telephone interpreting service is contacted and the doctor conducts the consultation with the patient using the service. For complicated consultations that are booked in advance, it is possible to arrange for an interpreter to be present.

Some receptionists say that there have been cases where a young child in the family acts as interpreter for older family members. You can see the problem that this could cause. There is also a danger that medical terminology can be incorrectly translated which could lead to serious problems (see Case Study 12).

Language barriers can also include deaf people who use signing to communicate. Signing is their first language, and they may have difficulty lip reading. In some services it is now possible to book a signer to attend an appointment, or the person brings their own signer.

Many of the issues related to barriers of access could be resolved if the service provider was aware of the particular needs of the client before making an appointment.

## CASE STUDY TWELVE:

In the 1970s a woman was having a baby in a London hospital and there were complications. The husband and wife spoke a particular dialect from the Asian sub-continent. The only person in the hospital who could be called upon to act as interpreter spoke a different dialect. The consultant said he wanted the patient and her husband to give a consent for a caesarean operation to save the child. The patient and her husband refused and the baby and mother died. In the inquiry that followed it was found that the interpreter had translated the word "caesarean" incorrectly as "sterilisation", and this is why the patient refused.

This would never happen nowadays, but even so, interpreting services in all aspects of care services are rather patchy. Although many health and social care services produce leaflets in different languages, there needs to be effective communication in the face to face situation

### Resource barriers

This is a key issue in health and social care services. Local services are dependent on national funding from central government. All services need to show that they are able to work within a budget, and provide "**best value**". This means cost effective services. Social services have to gain 7% of their income from charges they make to client groups. At the end of the financial year, budgets have to balance. A hospital trust cannot ask for more money if it overspends. It either has to carry the loss forward into the next year, or it has to cut services in order to stay within budget. Therefore, a ward may close or non-essential surgery may be cancelled.

Another key resource in health and care services is staff. At the moment there is a severe shortage of nursing and other staff in the NHS and in social care. One solution has been to recruit nurses from overseas, but this has its own problems.

*Postcode lottery (see Figure 2.30)*

Health authorities decide which drugs will be paid for and which will not be supported. Some drugs are very expensive and may have limited value. This can mean that different parts of the country may have different policies on paying for expensive drugs. One way of reducing this unfairness has been with the development of NICE (National Institute for Clinical Excellence). The role of NICE is to research new or expensive drugs and provide guidance as to whether the drug should be available on the NHS or not. NICE is also developing guidelines on referrals to hospital for conditions such as arthritis and skin complaints. It is hoped that by using national guidelines all patients will be treated fairly wherever they live in the UK.

## Activity

Can you think of ways to encourage more people into nursing, or to keep staff on in the NHS? In London, there is a plan to provide cheap housing for key workers in health and social care. Can you think of other ways to encourage workers?

---

**Figure 2.30** *The NHS postcode lottery*

# NHS postcode lottery 'worsened'

### By David Derbyshire – Medical Correspondent

The body set up to end the NHS postcode lottery has failed to improve the healthcare of patients, the drugs industry said yesterday.

Although NICE, the National Institute of Clinical Excellence, was intended to end confusion over drugs rationing, there are concerns that British patients are missing out on live-saving drugs available elsewhere in Europe. Many doctors wrongly used the existence of a NICE review into a drug as a reason not to prescribe it, the industry said.

In a separate attack, cancer charities said NICE was failing to listen to patients and called for a review into how drugs were appraised.

Evidence about "Nice blight" will be presented to MPs today by patient groups during a Health Select Commitee hearing. NICE was set up in 1998 to end the NHS drugs postcode lottery by advising on the cost effectiveness of new treatments.

Although the results of its appraisals are only recommendations, the Government promised that NICE would end regional differences in the availability of NHS treatments. But according to the Association of British Pharmaceutical Industry, NICE may have made things worse.

### Demand pressures

As more services develop, more people use them. One of the government's aims is to identify and support carers. At the moment many carers are unknown, but once they are identified and offered support this will put additional pressure on services in respite care for the cared for, as well as support services for the carers.

The increase in life expectancy means that the demand for services for older people has increased. One way of dealing with this is to encourage people to remain independent in their own homes, rather than use residential care or hospital services. However, staff are still needed to provide these services.

Increased demand for hip replacements in older people has led to government initiatives to speed up the process. Hip fractures are a common cause of hospital admission among older people. Prevention of accidents through exercise classes and safety checks in the home are additional programmes that have been developed.

### Rationing of services

Newspaper articles have identified the problems of inequality of access to services, including the prescribing of drugs. Different local authorities may have different priorities in offering certain services. As we have seen in the section on *Types of care services*, some services are offered at the discretion of the local authority, and the charges made for care services can vary across the UK. At the moment, Scotland is planning to provide free personal care to older people, but in the rest of the UK this will be charged for.

## Integration of services

With the *NHS Plan* (2000) and the *Care Standards Act* (2001) it is hoped that all health and care services will work more closely together in the future. The new PCTs (primary care trusts), social services, health trusts and the voluntary sector will be planning and delivering services locally. Because local professionals, who are aware of the needs of their area, will be working together, it is hoped that services will be more effective and clients will not be so confused about who is providing the service.

# THE MAIN JOBS IN HEALTH AND SOCIAL CARE AND EARLY YEARS SERVICES

What does care work involve and what skills do care practitioners need to perform their work roles?

Within the health and social care sectors, there are those staff who deliver care directly and those whose work is more indirectly involved with care.

Examples of direct care workers include: nurse, doctor, social worker, care assistant, nursery nurse.

Examples of indirect care workers include: clinic clerk, receptionist, cleaner.

## The difference between health care and social care

People who work as health workers usually look after patients who have health-related problems or conditions. People who work in social care are usually dealing with clients who have a range of personal and social needs.

## Activity

Look at the following examples of jobs and decide whether they are direct care or indirect care:
◗ hospital porter
◗ health visitor
◗ practice manager
◗ practice nurse
◗ chiropodist.
(Answers given on page 191.)

## Activity

Look at the following list of jobs and decide which is a health care job, and which is a social care job:
◗ health visitor
◗ district nurse
◗ dentist
◗ pharmacist
◗ social worker
◗ care assistant
◗ occupational therapist
◗ community psychiatric nurse
◗ housing officer.

Most of these jobs fit easily into either health care or social care. Two are problematic.

1. **Occupational therapists** are employed by social services to assess the needs of people in their homes and the physical support they may need (bath rails, commodes, walking aids). However, they can also be employed in hospitals to encourage people to develop practical skills and as part of therapeutic treatment of people with mental health problems.

2. The **community psychiatric nurse** is another example of a job that does not fit easily into either health or social care as, although the CPN has a nursing qualification, he or she also provides emotional support.

# OCCUPATIONAL AREAS IN HEALTH AND SOCIAL CARE

Before we start to look at the main jobs in health and social care, we need to be aware of the different sectors of employment.

The main categories are divided up as follows:

- medicine
- nursing
- community services
- social work
- child care
- professions allied to medicine (PAMS)
- administration and support work.

Within each of these groups, there tends to be a common core of training followed by specialist training. For example, all doctors follow a standard medical training and those who choose to specialise in general practice complete additional training. Hospital play specialists have usually completed their Diploma in nursery nursing before they complete the hospital play specialist course.

## Main jobs in health

### Medicine

Entry into medical school training is very competitive and applicants must have good grades at A level. The training lasts for five years. After training the doctor spends at least a year as a junior hospital doctor. After this period, doctors take additional training in order to become a specialist in their chosen area of practice.

## CASE STUDY THIRTEEN: SALMA

Salma is a GP in a busy South London practice. She is married with a young child. Salma took a specialist GP training course after her initial time as a junior doctor. She has a particular interest in paediatrics (children's medicine) and she attends the local children's hospital training sessions. She is also interested in recent developments in drugs and she is on the prescribing sub-committee of her local PCT Board. Salma has three partners at her practice, and she and her colleagues take it in turns to work on Saturdays.

Being a GP can be very demanding. Although many of the patients you see can have routine problems that are relatively easy to treat, you can also be faced with emergency situations that need instant decisions. Some patients may be extremely anxious, and some patients may be dying. It has been estimated that GPs can write up to 300 prescriptions a week and they can also see up to 20 people in one session at the surgery.

## Activity

Table 2.9 shows a list of qualities that a group of health and care workers identified as being essential for people working in health and social care. As you can see, personality traits and skills are listed, but the group also felt that these needed to be supported by knowledge. As a health or care worker you need to know **why** you do certain things.

Which 10 qualities would be most important in the role of the GP?

## Nursing as a career

At the moment, entry into the Diploma of Nursing requires applicants to have five GCSEs or the Advanced GNVQ in Health and Social Care or a similar award.

| PERSONAL QUALITIES | SKILLS |
|---|---|
| Sense of humour | Good communication skills: |
| Patient | ● verbal |
| Tactful | ● written |
| Sympathetic | ● non-verbal |
| Respect for others | Legible writing |
| Caring | Professional approach |
| Reliable | Observation skills |
| Punctual | Assessment skills |
| Good health | Listening skills |
| Flexible approach | Supervision of others |
| Polite | Record keeping |
| Willing to learn | IT skills |
| Shows initiative | Numeracy skills |
| Confident | Can work as part of a team |
| Can work under pressure | Can work independently |
| Friendly | Able to drive a car |
| Respects confidentiality | Good manual dexterity |
| Smart appearance | Telephone skills |
| Attention to hygiene | Attention to health and safety |
| Understanding of others | |
| Gets on with everyone | |

**UNDERPINNED BY KNOWLEDGE**

*Table 2.9  A range of qualities and skills identified by care workers*

Once students are accepted on to the Diploma, they follow a Common Foundation programme for one year and then they specialise in one of the following branches:

▶ Adult Nursing

▶ Mental Health

▶ Learning Disabilities

▶ Child Health.

Some students may decide they want to do the degree in nursing. Many nurses who are working in a hospital or in the community at the moment have completed additional training courses.

We will now look at some of the jobs in community nursing.

## CASE STUDY FOURTEEN: JOYCE

### The health visitor

Joyce is a health visitor attached to a busy health centre in South London.

This is a day in her working week:

| | |
|---|---|
| **9.00 am** | Arrive at the health centre. Check the post and any messages that have been left during the night. Phone and arrange visits to mothers of babies who have been discharged from the care of the midwife and are now Joyce's responsibility. |
| **10.00–12.00** | Child development clinic, advising mothers on diet and nutrition, sleeping problems. The details of all babies seen are logged on to the computer. |
| **12.00 pm** | Visit to local mother and baby hostel to advise mothers on baby care. This hostel is run by a local church for single unsupported girls. The girls go into the hostel when they are pregnant, and stay until the baby is six months old. During the visit Joyce advises on home safety, and weighs the babies on portable scales.<br><br>The lunch hour is spent dealing with phone calls, writing up reports, including referral to specialist. Although more work is done nowadays on computer, written records are still used. |
| **2.00 pm** | Joyce visits a woman of 75 who has urinary incontinence. During her visit Joyce takes the patient's medical history, number of pregnancies, and tests her urine. Joyce advises her how to avoid infections by drinking a lot of water, and she orders incontinence pads. Many women experience incontinence problems after the menopause. |
| **3.00 pm** | Joyce calls in on a new mother who has been discharged from the midwife. The health visitor takes over from the midwife on the tenth day. |
| **3.30 pm** | Joyce visits a family whose three-year-old daughter attended A & E with a suspected non-accidental injury. Joyce is the named health visitor at the health centre for these injuries, and she was contacted by the HV based at the hospital. |
| **7.30–9.00 pm** | Joyce runs the parentcraft class for women who are near the end of their pregnancy. Husbands or partners are encouraged to be present. |

During the evening she shows a video showing the birth of a baby, and demonstrates the development of the foetus and the delivery, using anatomical models and visual aids. The class is very lively, with people asking questions. In this part of the evening she organises the parents into groups and asks them to make a list of their worries about pregnancy and childbirth.

Do you think that Joyce needs different skills from the doctor.?
Look at the list again in Table 2.9 and decide which skills are important for Joyce.

### District nurses

District nurses are trained nurses involved with a wide range of patients. They visit people in their own homes to give clinical care and to advise on nursing aids and equipment. They will change dressings, give injections and administer other treatment. District nurses provide leadership and support to the nursing team. This may include working with health care assistants who are studying for their NVQ (National Vocational Qualification) and liaising with social services. Recent changes mean that district nurses are now able to prescribe drugs on a limited list once they have completed specialist training.

### Community psychiatric nurses

CPNs are employed by the Hospital and Community Mental Health Trust and are concerned with supporting people with mental health problems in the community. However, they often work closely with their colleagues in hospital.

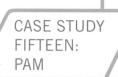

CASE STUDY
FIFTEEN:
PAM

Pam is a CPN in a busy suburban area. She belongs to a team of seven CPNs who are specialists in the care of patients with dementia. Although most of her patients are over 65, she also has younger patients who have been diagnosed as having dementia. Patients are referred to the consultant psychiatrist by their GPs. The psychiatrist sees them within a short time and then refers them to Pam and her team. Each CPN has a caseload of between 35 and 40 patients.

Pam sees her patients in their own home, and there are weekly team meetings to discuss the progress of patients and any problems.

Pam likes working in the community. She can work on her own initiative. She enjoys building up a relationship with the families she visits and seeing the progress of some of the patients. The challenges of the job include the stress caused by staff shortages, which can increase the workload; making difficult decisions; and doing the large amount of paperwork that is involved. It is also hard to say goodbye to patients when they have to go into residential care.

## Community pharmacist

Another important member of the community team is the community pharmacist (see Figure 2.31).

For simple complaints, such as coughs and colds, the pharmacist can offer advice.

With the development of NHS Direct, more people are being encouraged to talk to their pharmacist to discuss possible treatment. The pharmacist has a wide knowledge of drugs and can advise patients on the side effects they may experience when taking prescribed drugs. Pharmacists keep records of patients' prescriptions on computer so that they can refer to them.

Apart from giving advice and preparing prescriptions, the pharmacist may offer the following services:

▶ home delivery of drugs to housebound patients

▶ delivery of oxygen cylinders

▶ pregnancy testing

▶ some specialist blood testing for allergies through a private lab.

## Activity

We have now looked at several examples of jobs in the community. Are the qualities required for each job the same, or are they different?
Look again at Table 2.9 and think of the qualities that are needed for each of the jobs we have discussed in this section.

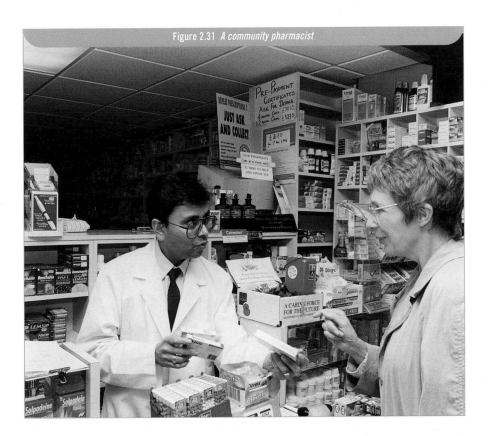

Figure 2.31 *A community pharmacist*

### Chiropodist

This is another member of the community team. Chiropodists are concerned with maintaining healthy feet. Although many chiropodists are private, self-employed practitioners, NHS chiropodists are attached to health centres and can be accessed by referral from a GP or nurse, or by self-referral. Certain groups of people are especially prone to foot problems, such as older people or people with diabetes. The chiropodist can treat infections of the nails and feet, and advise on foot care.

### Dentist

Dentists have a long period of training before they are qualified. Like doctors, the training takes five years and dentists continue to have regular training once they are in practice, as many of the procedures change and they need to keep up to date. Some dentists have their own private practices, but most dentists have a mixture of NHS and private patients.

Apart from fillings, replacing broken and damaged teeth and cosmetic dentistry, some dentists specialise in orthodontics, when they treat crooked teeth with appliances that can be fixed or removable. Dentists advise patients about hygiene and dental care.

### Dental nurse

A dental nurse has to have at least five GCSEs to be accepted for training. Once qualified, the dental nurse continues to attend training sessions to adapt his/her knowledge. Modern Apprenticeship Schemes are bing developed in dental nursing.

## CASE STUDY SIXTEEN: SIOBHAN

Siobhan is a dental nurse in a busy practice in the South of England. Her day is as follows.

I am in the surgery shortly after 8 am, preparing for the treatment for the day. The first appointment is at 8.30. The day can be very varied, from a straightforward filling to complicated bridge work, and I have to make sure that the dentist has everything he needs.

As well as mixing the materials for fillings and dental impressions, I assist with taking X-rays and reassuring patients. I still go to training courses to keep up to date with changes. I have been at this surgery for ten years now, so I know a lot of the patients and their families. The most enjoyable part of the job is that every day is different, and I feel I am really using my skills. We see everyone, from young children having their first check up, to women who are expecting babies, and older people.

The work can be quite tiring and I am pleased to put my feet up at the end of the day. It is nice having the weekends free.

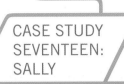

**CASE STUDY SEVENTEEN: SALLY**

Sally is a staff nurse on a busy medical ward of 28 beds. Sally returned to nursing recently, having had two children. Once they were at secondary school, Sally decided she wanted to go back to nursing, so she approached her local hospital who arranged for her to go on a retraining course for 12 weeks. During this time, Sally spent time on different wards, and at the end of the retraining she was offered part-time work. She works four days a week from 7.30 am to 4 pm. When she arrives on the ward in the morning, she receives the report from the night staff and uses the computer to log in the names of patients in the ward. Many records are now kept on computer, although patients also have written notes. During the day Sally gives out medicines, gives injections, changes dressings, talks to relatives, admits new patients, and deals with emergency situations which could include coping with a patient whose heart stops beating and needs resuscitation.

Sally also teaches procedures to student nurses. At the moment the ward is divided into sections for men and women, and because of this layout there is a great deal of walking. Sally enjoys the pace of work and the variety of work – every day is different. The stresses of the job include being short staffed, never having enough time to spend time with patients and relatives, and the endless paperwork.

### Nursing in hospital

Nursing posts in hospital can be in surgical or medical settings, in out-patients or in mental health care.

After you have completed your GCSE course, you may think about becoming a health care assistant in a hospital. Figure 2.32 gives a job description of a HCA in a busy London hospital. Look at it and decide what skills are required.

## Jobs in social care

Figure 2.34 shows the range of jobs that are available in social work. At the moment, qualified social workers have to take a two-year diploma course or a degree in social work. The qualifications are currently being reviewed, and all qualifying programmes are likely to take three years in future.

## Activity

Case studies 17 and 18 give examples of different nursing posts. Look at these and decide which skills are needed.

Figure 2.32 *Job description of a health care assistant*

## Greenlands Hospital Trust

### Job Description: Health Care Assistant

**Functions**

*Patient care*

1. Help with nursing care as instructed by nursing staff, including bathing, bed making, lifting patients and help with meals as necessary.
2. Caring for patients' personal clothing and other property in accordance with agreed policies relating to security and confidentiality.
3. Cleaning of beds and cleaning of lockers.

*Ward responsibilities*

1. Assisting the nursing staff to keep the ward tidy, including equipment and treatment rooms.
2. Assisting in checking, unpacking and storing of items delivered to the ward.
3. Answering the telephone and taking messages as required.
4. Being familiar with procedures related to health and safety, fire and other emergencies.

*General*

1. Observing complete confidentiality of information and records at all times, both on and off site.
2. Complying with all the Trust policies as they relate to staff, patients, relatives and visitors.
3. Undertaking errands as required.
4. Maintaining good working relations amongst staff.
5. Establishing and maintaining good relations with visitors and relatives, helping them to find their way around the hospital site.

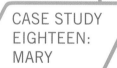

CASE STUDY
EIGHTEEN:
MARY

**Nursing team leader for mental health**

Mary Andrews (Figure 2.33) trained as a Registered Mental Nurse, and has specialised in mental health in hospital ever since. She is responsible for a team of 23 nursing staff. The nurses are trained staff like Mary, and also NVQ nursing assistants. She is in charge of 181 mental health beds. These include secure wards (which are kept locked), acute wards (where people may have tried to commit suicide), and long-stay wards for people with dementia.

Mary works five days a week, but is also on a rota for on-call duties at weekends and nights. She attends a lot of meetings with community nurses and voluntary organisations who are caring for people in the community with mental health problems. Mary is employed by the Hospital and Community Mental Health Trust. She enjoys her job and describes it as challenging. Every day is different and she never knows what emergency she will deal with next. It can be stressful working with anxious relatives and also with people with violent or challenging behaviour, but Mary would not want to do anything else.

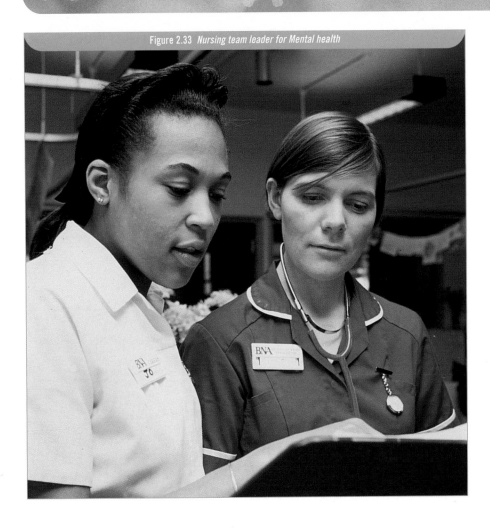

Figure 2.33 *Nursing team leader for Mental health*

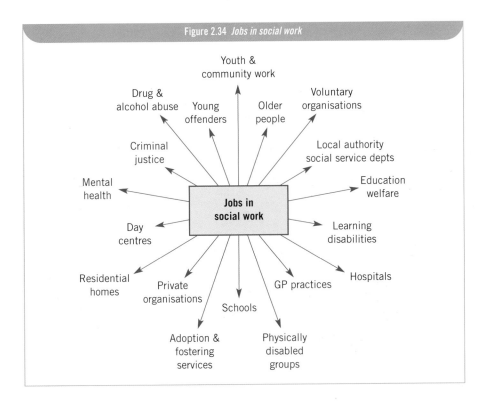

Figure 2.34 *Jobs in social work*

Most professional social workers are employed as **field** social workers. This means they work in the community or institution and have certain client groups. If you turn back to Figure 2.17 on page 88 showing the structure of the typical social services department, you can see that social workers are attached to a range of client groups, families and children, people with mental health problems, people with learning disabilities, etc.

Social workers can be employed in private organisations or by voluntary groups.

Social workers also work in hospitals, and this often involves liaising with other local council services for people returning home.

## CASE STUDY NINETEEN: DEBBIE

Debbie is a social worker, employed by a Social Services Department, in the Children Services section (see Figure 2.35). Debbie is responsible for following up incidents of non-accidental injury that have been reported by the local A & E department. Each day Debbie sees children and families and makes an assessment of their needs. She may provide them with advice or counselling, or put them in touch with other agencies that may be able to help them, such as Child Psychiatry for family problems or Social Security for financial assistance.

Although Debbie works 9 to 5, Monday to Friday, she is also on call some weekends and evenings. Apart from doing initial assessments, Debbie may help some families over a longer period of time with problems such as money, housing or relationship problems. She will attend regular case conferences for children who have been identified as 'at risk' by Social Services. In these meetings she will discuss the family with the other professionals involved and make a child protection plan to keep the children safe. The focus is on supporting and helping families care for their children properly. It is only in very exceptional circumstances, when a child has suffered significant harm, that she would apply to the court to take the child into care. When she does this, she has to prove to the court that the Social Services could do a better job of looking after the child than the family.

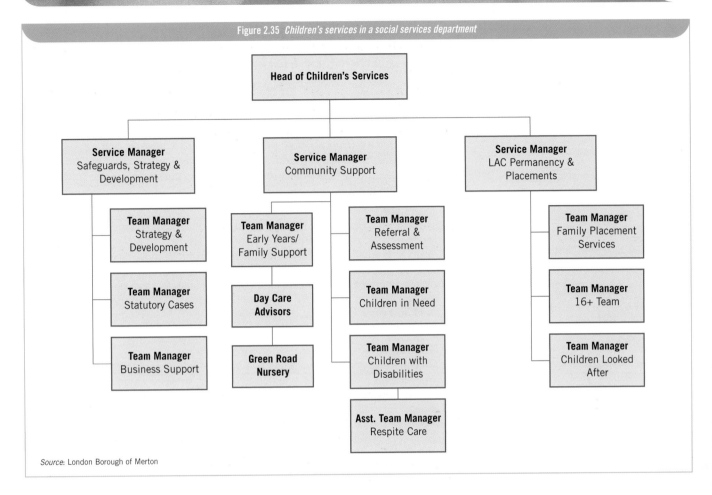

**Figure 2.35** *Children's services in a social services department*

*Source*: London Borough of Merton

## Social care

Social care workers can include people with NVQs (National Vocational Qualifications) and other qualifications and also unqualified people. They often work under the supervision of the social worker or qualified nurse. Social care jobs are usually found in three main areas:

▶ domiciliary care (people being looked after in their own homes)

▶ residential care

▶ day care.

Figure 2.36 is the job description of a home carer, a person who looks after people in their own homes.

Job descriptions tend to focus on tasks that the worker has to do, but as we will see in a later section of this chapter, a care worker has to carry out these tasks taking account of the individual needs of the client.

### Activity

What skills are needed in this job? (See Table 2.9)

Figure 2.36 *Job description of a home care worker*

# Department of Housing and Social Services
## Post: Home Carer

*General Purpose of the Job*
To provide seven day personal care and domestic help to people living in their own homes. Service users will be older people, families with children, and people with a disability or mental illness, including those with carers such as relatives or friends. The post-holder will be a team member committed to providing a caring service which puts the user first.

*Personal Care*
1. Assist with day to day grooming, washing, bathing (parker bath only) and dressing, getting the user up and putting to bed.
2. Help with toileting, dealing with incontinence and catheter care, emptying and disinfecting commodes.
3. Assist with feeding, including preparation of meals and awareness of special dietary needs.
4. Administration of medication prescribed by the doctor, including applying creams and inserting eye drops.

*Domestic duties – to be discussed and agreed with client*
1. To undertake general housework, bed making and changing bed linen.
2. Washing personal clothing and household linen in user's home or local laundrette, or day centre.
3. Shop, pay bills, collect prescriptions and pensions.
4. Assist with financial affairs, keeping accurate records of all transactions.
5. Help with correspondence and letter writing.
6. Assist with pets.

*General duties*
1. Write detailed reports on user's progress and changes in their needs, behaviour or circumstances on a care plan in the user's home. To inform the team leader of any such changes.
2. Attend training sessions and meetings such as team meetings, case conferences and supervision sessions as required.
3. Be responsible and handle emergencies with users in non-office hours which may require the carer to make a decision to call medical or emergency aid.
4. Liaise with other professional involved with the user, e.g. GP, social worker, care manager, warden.
5. Accompany the user to pre-arranged appointments and occasional shopping trips, outings as required.
6. Carers may hold keys for their users and must be responsible for their safe keeping.
7. To establsh a relationship with the user, give support to those under stress and provide companionship and a link with the community.
8. Work in accordance with department policies, practice and legislation relevant to their work, in particular, Health and Safety at Work and complaints.
9. Must carry out all duties in accordance with the Council's Equal Opportunities Policy.
10. Any other comparable duties required by the Line Manager.

## Caring for Children

Workers in child care may have a range of qualifications. Figure 2.37 shows the main jobs looking after children.

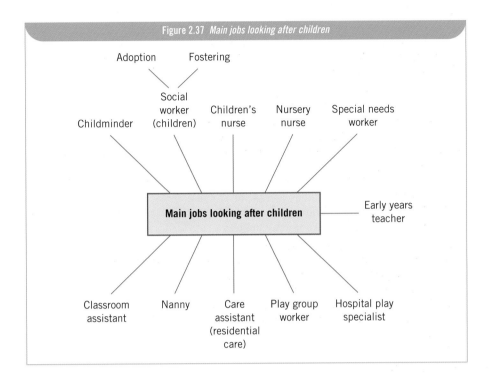

**Figure 2.37** *Main jobs looking after children*

## Activity

In pairs, interview someone who works with children, either in a school, nursery, hospital or as a nanny. Ask them what qualifications and skills they need for the job. What do they do each day in their job? What are the good things and bad things about their job? Discuss your findings with the rest of your group.

Figure 2.38 shows the job description of a nursery nurse working in a crèche attached to a hospital. What skills are required for this post?

## Professions allied to Medicine (PAMS)

In addition to medicine and nursing, there are a number of roles within the health care occupational area (see Table 2.10).

Figure 2.38 *Job description of a nursery nurse*

**Job Description: Nursery Nurse in the hospital crèche**

*Role*
1. To be directly responsible for the general wellbeing of the children in the crèche and to satisfy their basic needs.
2. To carry out all professional duties as you may be required to do.
3. To maintain health and safety standards at all times.

*Duties*
1. To organise play facilities and to act in a caring role, i.e. changing, feeding and the care of clothing.
2. To ensure that any child who appears in any way unwell is removed from the crèche as soon as possible by the parent (or other responsible person nominated by the parent) and that the crèche manager is informed.
3. To discuss with the manager any child who is causing, or appears to have problems.
4. To see that the toys and play equipment are maintained in good order. That any faulty or potentially dangerous equipment is made immediately inaccessible to the children, and its condition reported to the most senior member of staff.
5. To be responsible for ordering toys and play equipment and at Christmas to assist with the selection and distribution of toys.
6. To be responsible for the overall tidiness and appearance of the crèche and to contribute to the general decorations.
7. To take the children for walks and other activities as appropriate, provided that permission is given by the parents.

*Education and training*
1. To assist in the instruction of all work experience students.
2. To maintain an up to date knowledge of developments in nursery nursing. This may include attending courses after discussion with the manager.

*Safety*
1. To be conversant with procedures carried out in case of accident.
2. To be conversant with procedures carried out in case of fire.

Examples of PAMS include the following:

▶ speech and language therapist

▶ occupational therapist

▶ radiographer

▶ radiotherapist.

These qualifications all require a three-year degree course at university, but there are also opportunities for people to work as assistants to these workers.

| JOB TITLE | QUALIFICATIONS | CLIENT GROUP | JOB ROLE |
|---|---|---|---|
| Dietitian | Degree | All ages. Healthy living centres/hospitals/ community. | Promotion of healthy eating. Diets for specific illnesses/problems – obesity, diabetes, metabolic disorders. |
| Occupational therapist | Degree | All ages. Working hospitals /community. People with learning disabilities, physical disabilities. Mobility problems. Mental health problems. | Promote independent living and prevent disability. Recommend and supply equipment and aids to support patients' lifestyles. |
| Optometrist | Degree | All ages, especially children. People with visual problems. | Perform eye tests, and prescribe corrective lenses. Identify medical conditions such as glaucoma and retinal problems. |
| Pharmacist | Degree | All ages, especially older people/families. Work in hospitals and community. | Advise on drugs to doctors/ patients. Advise patients on how to treat minor conditions. |
| Physiotherapist | Degree | All ages, especially people after operations, and in rehabilitation. Work in community and hospital. | Support and treat people who have illness, accidents or problems caused by ageing. Exercises/treatment to restore and develop the function of the body. |
| Radiographer (Diagnostic) | Degree | All ages. Usually work in hospitals. Can be diagnosing illness/disease. | Record and produce images by a range of processes to identify disease and extent of injuries. |
| Speech and language therapist | Degree | All ages, people who have trouble with communication and/or swallowing difficulties. | Assist carers and other health workers to support people with problems, using exercises and techniques to improve speech (stroke) and swallowing (dysfunction) |
| Chiropodist (podiatrist) | Degree | All ages, children, adults, older people with foot problems. | Maintain healthy feet. Assess, diagnose and treat foot conditions, veruccae, minor surgery in some cases. |

Table 2.10 Professions allied to medicine

## CASE STUDY TWENTY: PAT

Community physiotherapist

Not all physios work in hospital. Pat works as a community physio in Devon. Here is a day from her diary.

**7.00 am** Get up.

**8.10 am** Leave for work.

**8.30 am** Arrive at the local hospital for a team meeting with the hospital physio to discuss patients who will be discharged home and need support. Catch up with paperwork and telephone/fax messages.

**9.30 am** First visit – a blind patient who walked into a ditch and broke her leg. The plaster has been removed. She needs to have physio to regain her muscle power and must do exercises.

**10.00 am** Visit to nursing home to visit two patients. Malcolm is returning home and needs instructions and exercises on walking using a stick. Moyra has a chest infection, so she needs help to improve her breathing and general mobility.

**11.30 am** Visit to Mrs Stewart who has been discharged from hospital and is finding it difficult to cope. Pat asks the occupational therapist to visit and assess her needs and what additional aids that might help her.

**12.30 pm** To hospital to write up notes. Pat has to keep one set of handwritten notes for her own use, one set on the computer, and the patient has hand-held records that are kept in their home. (sandwich lunch)

**1.45 pm** Ward visit with Jan (physio assistant) to check on post-operative patients.

**2.30 pm** Home visit to Brian who has a muscular wasting disease, for breathing exercises, passive exercises of limbs and massage.

**3.20. pm** Visit to remote farm (Pat has trouble finding it). The farmer, John, has had a stroke. His wife is having difficulty bathing him so Pat refers him to the occupational therapist for advice. Pat spends some time talking to John's wife about how to support her husband.

As you can see from this example, working in the community, especially in remote areas, can require different skills. People in the country may be quite isolated and visits from health care professionals are not just concerned with clinical matters, but are seen as a way to feel part of the community. Pat sees fewer patients in a day than physios in hospital, but the relationship between patient and therapist can be very different and require different skills. Additional skills that Pat needs are the ability to read a map, and to drive!

So far, we have looked at jobs that give direct care to patients in the community and in the hospital, but there are several workers in GP practices who give support to doctors and nurses.

## Practice managers

These are key people in the practice, and are in charge of the receptionists, secretaries and other workers. They have overall responsibility for the smooth running of the surgery. They make sure that the computers are working, and make appointments for drug representatives to see the doctors. They ensure that all staff working in the practice are aware of health and safety issues. They interview new staff and provide an induction to the practice. They are responsible for the holiday rota system, and they deal with complaints from patients.

Practice managers have a wide range of backgrounds. They could have previous experience in social care or nursing, but they have to have good office skills. In order to become a practice manager, you have to take the Diploma in Practice Management.

## Receptionist

A receptionist is the first person the patient comes into contact with when entering the surgery or when phoning with a query or to make an appointment. Many patients are very anxious when they call on the receptionist. The receptionist must be careful to be aware of issues of confidentiality. If a patient telephones the surgery wanting to know the result of a test, there are usually clear guidelines about the correct procedure to be followed and the doctor will usually speak to the patient personally if there is an

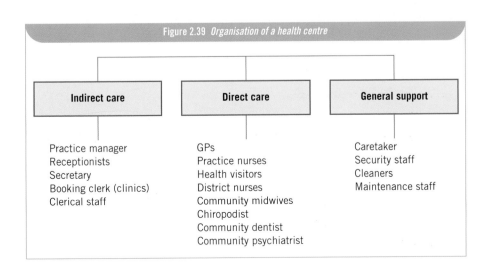

Figure 2.39 *Organisation of a health centre*

| Indirect care | Direct care | General support |
| --- | --- | --- |
| Practice manager | GPs | Caretaker |
| Receptionists | Practice nurses | Security staff |
| Secretary | Health visitors | Cleaners |
| Booking clerk (clinics) | District nurses | Maintenance staff |
| Clerical staff | Community midwives | |
| | Chiropodist | |
| | Community dentist | |
| | Community psychiatrist | |

abnormal result. Receptionists may hear details of a private nature being discussed, and it is very important that these matters are not referred to elsewhere.

Figure 2.39 shows the organisation of a health centre.

# EFFECTIVE COMMUNICATION SKILLS

The health and social care worker must be able to communicate effectively with a wide range of patients or clients:

- babies/children
- adolescents
- young adults
- older people
- other health workers
- doctors
- nurses
- teachers
- police
- social workers.

Lack of effective communication between the care worker and the patient will mean that the client will not receive the support they need.

Communication can take many forms. We will look at alternative forms of communication for people with specific problems later in the chapter. In this section we will be looking at communication in the form of:

- verbal communication
- non-verbal communication
- written communication.

## Verbal communication

Everyone says they know how to talk, but in health and social care it is important to use verbal communication effectively when:

- assessing patients
- identifying needs

▶ giving information

▶ encouraging patients to express their own views and be independent.

## Questions

Most health and social workers use questions every day.

There are several types of question.

1 **Closed questions**, for example: How old are you? What is your name? Are you married?

These questions are appropriate when brief factual material is needed, but they do not encourage conversation and expression of thoughts and feelings.

2 **Open (or open-ended) questions**. These give an opportunity for fuller, deeper answers, e.g. How do you feel about moving into sheltered housing? Is there anything you need to know about how to breast feed the baby? **How**, **what**, **feel** and **think** are useful words for encouraging a full response.

3 **Biased questions**. These indicate the answer the questioner wants or expects to hear, e.g. You have settled into the routine of the home, haven't you? It isn't necessary to go over your medication again, is it?

4 **Multiple questions**. These include more than one question and can cause confusion, e.g. Is this a serious problem, when did it start? How did the accident happen, what did you do?

It is the responsibility of the health and social care worker to make sure that communication is effective.

## Barriers to communication

**Communication is a two way process**. We all communicate every day. Think about a typical day in your life and the communications that take place.

You may have identified some of the following:

▶ informal conversation with friends, either one to one or else in a group

▶ more formal discussions at work or college

▶ telephone conversations, formal and informal

▶ letters from friends, emails, faxes.

All these forms of communication use words, either spoken or written.

## Activity

Which of the following questions are closed, open, biased, or multiple?

1. How are you?
2. How often do you come to the surgery?
3. Have you collected your repeat prescriptions, which ones do you have?
4. You prefer to do your own shopping don't you?

Think about a recent communication that went well. Why did it go well?

Now think about a recent communication that left you feeling awkward, angry, or frustrated. What was the problem?

**Barriers to communication can include the following**:

▶ insufficient information is given

▶ the environment is unhelpful – noisy, lack of privacy, too many people talking at the same time

▶ the other person does not seem interested in what you have to say

▶ lack of understanding due to language used.

## Listening skills

Listening skills are very important in health and social care. In ordinary conversations there tends to be a pattern to conversation, e.g. Mary tells Surinder about what she did on Saturday night, and Surinder tells Mary what she did on Saturday night. We can see that there is an exchange of information. In effective listening the pattern is different. In effective listening you need to concentrate on the feelings of the other person and put your own views and feelings to one side.

Look at the following conversation:

*Jane:* I feel very tired. I suppose it is my age; everything seems to be such an effort.

*Practice nurse:* Yes, the "change" is not fun is it? I have awful night sweats and shout at the family.

What is the problem with the practice nurse's response?

You can see that the nurse is more concerned with expressing her own feelings, rather than listening effectively to Jane.

Listening effectively can be developed through the method called **reflecting back**. The care worker checks that they are fully understanding what the client is saying by restating what has been said. This helps the client to make their feelings clear. Reflecting back is used only in the discussion of feelings, not in other situations.

Read this example of reflecting back:

*Mother:* I just feel so useless. I never realised having a baby was such hard work. I seem to run about all day and I never get the place straight, and I feel so tired.

*Health Visitor:* Why do you think you feel so tired?

*Mother:* I suppose I feel I want everything to be perfect. My mother-in-law lives nearby. She is always popping in. Her house always looks perfect. She must think I am useless.

*Health Visitor:* Why do you think your mother-in-law thinks you are useless?

*Mother:* She has never approved of me, and it is even worse now.

*Health Visitor:* Do you think it has got worse since you had the baby?

By reflecting back in this way, the health worker may be able to help the patient identify the real problem. In this case, the problem may be the relationship between the two women, rather than the birth of the new baby. On the other hand, it could be that the mother has postnatal depression. In either case, effective listening is a useful tool in helping people to understand their feelings.

Communication skills do not just include listening and talking, but they also include non-verbal communication.

## Activity

1.  Working with a partner, move your chairs so you are sitting back to back. Without turning round, take it in turns to talk to each other, one acting as speaker, the other acting as listener. The one acting as listener is not allowed to say anything, and that includes grunting and laughing. When you have finished, discuss how you felt, as a listener and as a talker.

2.  Sitting face to face, take it in turns to act as listener and talker. This time the listener avoids looking at the speaker during their conversation.
    How does this feel?

# Non-verbal communication

**Non-verbal communication is communication without words.** The following are examples of non-verbal communication:

- physical contact – touching, holding hands, hugging, etc
- proximity – how close you sit or stand when you are talking to people
- posture – how you stand or sit, crossed arms, crossed legs, leaning forward
- gestures – what you do with your hands and arms, also nodding or shaking your head
- facial expression – smiling, laughing, frowning
- eye contact and movement – staring, blinking, winking, looking at someone
- tone of voice – loud, soft, aggressive,
- pace of voice – speaking fast, slowly, hesitating.

The reasons why you found the first exercise uncomfortable in the activity is that we look at the person we are talking to in order to gain a response, and we can respond using non-verbal communication as well to reinforce the communication process.

The second exercise also demonstrates the importance of eye contact when communicating with someone.

Look at Figure 2.40. This shows a photograph of Philip, a volunteer worker, talking to a client at a day centre. Make a list of non-verbal communication you can see.

Philip is looking at Mrs Tate; he is smiling and he is sitting in his chair at the same level at Mrs Tate. Another interesting thing we can see here, is that Philip is reflecting Mrs Tate's facial expressions.

This is called mirroring, and is often done unconsciously when people are trying to establish an equal relationship.

Next time you are in a bar, or in the college dining room, make a note of the non-verbal communication you can see occurring between two people. Not only may you see facial expressions mirrored, but you may see other gestures reflected by the couples, such as touching their own hair, hand movements, etc. We need to be aware of non-verbal communication, and also how some forms of verbal communication may be appropriate in some situations and not in others.

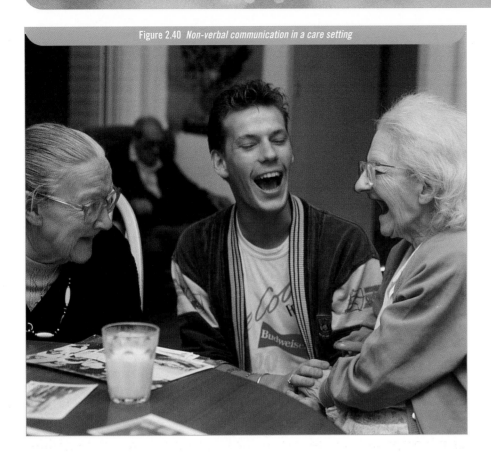

Figure 2.40 *Non-verbal communication in a care setting*

## Physical contact

Health and social care workers often touch patients and clients in order to show support and understanding. Look at Figure 2.41. The photograph shows Ashna, a volunteer at a day centre, with a client. Note the non-verbal communication that is shown by all the people in the photograph. You can see that Ashna is holding Mrs Gibson's hand. Why do you think she is doing this? Would you think it was appropriate if Ashna was a male carer? As care workers we need to be aware of the appropriate use of touch, especially on different parts of the body. The hands and arms are usually seen as acceptable areas to touch, but to touch other parts of the body, such as thigh, neck or knee, would be seen as off-limits unless you are massaging or washing someone. Again, there are cultural differences. Asian women would not wish to be touched by a man. Because of problems of accusations of abuse, all care workers need to be aware of the appropriate use of touch.

We have discussed communication – now it is your turn to practise your own communication skills.

Figure 2.41 *Using non-verbal communication*

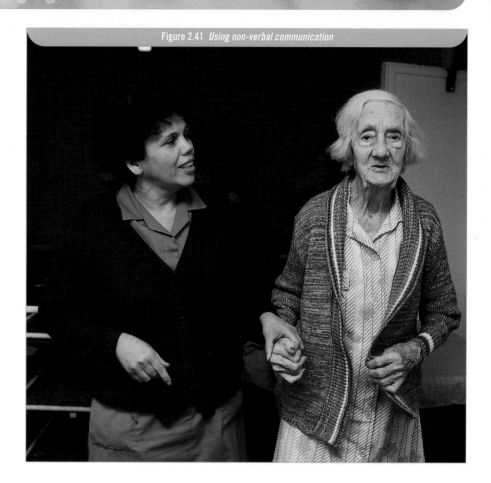

# Activity

Working in groups or pairs, try the following role plays.

1. You are the receptionist in a busy GP Practice. Mrs Hall telephones you and demands an immediate appointment with the doctor. Mrs Hall starts the conversation by saying, 'I really must see the doctor today,,' in an aggressive tone of voice. How do you deal with this?

2. You are working in the A & E department on a Friday night. A man who has been waiting for two hours comes over to you and starts being very aggressive about the delay. You suspect he has been drinking.

3. Working on the maternity unit, you answer the phone. A male voice asks how Charlotte Spencer is. Charlotte is a teenager who is having a difficult pregnancy and her mother is her next of kin. How do you respond to the caller? (Remember to be careful about confidentiality.)

4. You are a care worker in a residential home. You know Mr Patel is a diabetic and you see him eating some chocolates that have been given to the home. What do you say?

5.  You are an occupational therapist making a home assessment on Mrs Khan's mobility in her home. You need to assess how well she will cope at home after a recent operation. You notice frayed carpets and trailing flexes in the living room that may cause an accident. How do you start the conversation?

6.  You are a dental nurse and as part of your role you have to advise patients on how to clean their teeth properly. How might you change your approach for:
    ▶ a young child
    ▶ a teenager
    ▶ an older man
    ▶ a pregnant woman.

As you can see in all six cases, it isn't just the words you say that are important, but tone of voice, posture, facial expression, and gestures. On the phone, the tone of voice is very important, and you also have to speak more clearly and slowly as the person you are speaking to cannot see you for additional non-verbal information.

If you become impatient or aggressive with an aggressive patient or client, the situation can get worse, so it is important to keep calm before you say anything.

**Useful strategies**:

▶ If something isn't clear, ask for additional information. Sometimes this slows down the communication and can reduce tension.

▶ Take a deep breath and speak slowly and clearly.

▶ Maintain eye contact if face to face, and try to sit down rather than stand up, as people are more relaxed if they are sitting down. If the patient is in bed or in a chair, make sure you are at the same level, rather than standing over them.

▶ Respect issues of confidentiality.

▶ Don't try to score points or put people down.

## Benefits of effective communication

▶ The care worker can obtain and provide useful information that is relevant to clients'/patients' well being.

▶ It enables the care worker to support and understand the client/patient.

▶ It assists teamwork.

▶ It can help patients make their needs known.

If communication is **not effective**:

▶ patients can feel angry and resentful

▶ patients feel they are not being listened to and understood

▶ patients don't understand why certain procedures are happening

▶ patients may not follow treatment and exercise that may help them recover.

We will be looking at certain groups with specific communication problems later in the chapter.

## Written communication

In health and social care work, written communication is very important.

Your list could include:

▶ patient records

▶ care plans

▶ referral letters

▶ accident report forms

▶ prescriptions

▶ consent forms.

Patients' records are legal documents and could be used in a court of law. It is important they are:

▶ clear

▶ easy to read

▶ concise

▶ based on fact and not on opinion.

Consider these two examples of a patient record of Mrs Brown who is on the medical ward.

### Example A

Mrs Brown had a good night.

### Example B

Mrs Brown slept for six hours without medication. She woke up at 6 am and said she was free from pain, and did not require a pain killer.

### Discussion

In Example A, 'a good night,' could mean anything. It is vague and does not give any information.

## Activity

Make a list of written communication used in health and social care.

In Example B, we know that Mrs Brown slept for six hours, she was not in pain, and did not need a painkiller. The use of Mrs Brown's own words is also seen as a reliable record.

## Other forms of communication

Other forms of communication used in health and social care can include:

▶ posters (often to do with health promotion)

▶ leaflets

▶ diagrams.

When communicating with children, leaflets may be too complicated, and diagrams may be more appropriate.

Figure 2.42 is an example of a record kept by a child who is attending an enuresis clinic (for bedwetting). The child colours in the appropriate box. It is clear and gives an encouraging message to the child. It is also easy for the nurse to check the progress that is being made.

**Figure 2.42 Example of a child-friendly chart**

# WEEK 1

| | | | | | remarks |
|---|---|---|---|---|---|
| MON | | | | | |
| TUE | | | | | |
| WED | | | | | |
| THU | | | | | |
| FRI | | | | | |
| SAT | | | | | |
| SUN | | | | | |

# PRINCIPLES OF GOOD PRACTICE AND THE CARE VALUE BASE

The **care value base** underpins the work of everyone in health, social care and early years services. The value base underpins all training in care. It is used as the basis for NVQs (National Vocational Qualifications) in acute care in hospitals, and care in residential homes, nurseries and domiciliary work.

Care practitioners use guidelines and codes of practice to empower clients by:

- promoting anti-discriminatory practice
- maintaining confidentiality of information
- promoting individuals' rights to dignity, independence, health and safety
- acknowledging individuals' personal beliefs and identity
- protecting individuals from abuse
- promoting effective communication and relationships
- providing individualised care.

## Promoting anti-discriminatory practice

Discrimination occurs very frequently. **Discrimination** means that certain people are treated less favourably than others because of a personal characteristic they have. Certain groups are more likely to experience discrimination. These are:

- people with learning disabilities
- older people
- people with physical disabilities
- people with mental health problems
- women
- minority ethnic groups
- minority religious groups
- gay men and lesbians.

Discrimination may be direct or indirect.

## Direct discrimination

If a landlord puts a notice in the window for a lodger that reads 'No Irish or Blacks,' you can see that this is a clear example of discrimination, with certain groups being treated unfairly. To write a notice like this would be illegal nowadays.

An example of direct discrimination would be a clear statement of different treatment for a certain group. Direct discrimination of certain groups is banned by law.

## Indirect discrimination

What do you think of this advertisement?

You could say that this is an example of indirect discrimination, because although the advert doesn't clearly state that it wants white males, the personal factors required make this likely. Not many women are 6 foot tall, and workers who have English as a second language are less likely to have GCSE at the standard stated.

If the advertiser was challenged over this advert, he/she would need to prove that the height and English qualification were essential requirements of the job.

At the moment, age discrimination is not covered by legislation.

> **Cook wanted for nursing home.**
>
> Must be strong, 6 foot tall and have a good standard of English, preferably GCSE at A to C.

## Legislation

The main Acts of Parliament that are relevant to discrimination are:

▶ **The Race Relations Act (1976)**

This Act bans all forms of racial discrimination in work, housing and the provision of services. The Act has been revised to include indirect discrimination (Race Relations Amendment Act 2000).

▶ **The Sex Discrimination Act (1975)**

This Act provides equal rights to men and women in work, services and access to facilities. The Act covers both direct and indirect discrimination.

▶ **Disability Discrimination Act (1995)**

This Act gives rights to disabled people in employment, access to education and transport, housing and obtaining goods and services. However, although the legislation exists there are examples where indirect discrimination occurs.

▶ **Human Rights Act (1998)**

This Act covers a range of human rights that may affect health and care practice in the future. The following Articles are the most relevant:

*Article 2* – Everyone's life shall be protected by law.

*Article 3* – No-one should be subjected to torture or to inhuman or degrading treatment or punishment.

*Article 5* – Everyone has the right to liberty and security of their person.

*Article 6* – Everyone is entitled to a fair and public hearing in any civil or criminal matter.

*Article 8* – Everyone has the right to respect for their private and family life, their home and correspondence.

*Article 9* – Everyone has the right to freedom of thought, conscience and religion.

*Article 10* – Everyone has the right to freedom of expression.

*Article 12* – Men and women of marriageable age have the right to marry and have a family.

*Article 14* – The enjoyment of rights and freedoms should be secured without discrimination on any grounds such as sex, race, colour, language, religion, political or other opinion, national or social origin, association with a national minority, property, birth or other status.

# Activity

Look at the following care issues and identify which Article is most relevant (in some instances there could be more than one possibility).

1. Peter, who has Downs Syndrome, lives in sheltered accommodation. If he wants to withdraw money from his bank account he has to have the signature of his key worker.
2. Maria, who has a mild learning disability, wants to start living with her boyfriend.
3. Craig has a disagreement over the level of care he is receiving. His GP decides he wants to remove him from his list of patients.
4. Surita, who is a wheelchair user, wants to have a baby, but when she talks about this to her care worker, she is discouraged.
5. Richard has a long-standing mental health problem. He has a crisis and he is admitted to hospital as a compulsory patient (this is called **sectioning**). It is decided he needs to have an ECT (Electro-Convulsive Therapy) and also heavy sedation.
6. A recent report in a local paper highlights the widespread use of tranquillisers in nursing homes to keep patients quiet and easy to deal with.

As you can see, the *Human Rights Act* links into the value base and may have an important effect on the way health and care issues are resolved in the future.

Look at this extract from the future prescribing plan from a health authority:

*'It is not expected that prescriptions for this drug will be given to people over 75'.*

This would appear to be an example of discrimination on the basis of age.

The organisation Age Concern has collected evidence that older people may not be offered treatment and services because of their age (see Figure 2.43).

Other examples of discriminatory practice in health and social care could include the following:

▶ a nurse who applies for promotion but is rejected because she is taking drugs to control her epilepsy

▶ a nursery that refuses to take a child with HIV

▶ a nursery that refuses to take a child who has a facial disfigurement, saying it will frighten the other children

▶ a teenager with Downs Syndrome who cannot find a dentist willing to take him on his list

▶ a refugee who cannot find a GP to take him on as a patient.

People are treated unfairly because of prejudice and the use of stereotypes that are often reinforced by the media.

For example, the stereotype of older people is that they are all deaf and act like children.

Figure 2.43 *Ageism*

# Ageist health barriers
### *Restore clinical need as the NHS gateway*

Earlier this year a Gallup poll of 1,600 people over 50 found 1 in 20 felt they had been refused treatment on the grounds of their age – and 1 in 10 (almost 2m people if extrapolated nationwide) felt they had been treated differently since hitting 50. Age Concern, the pressure group which commissioned the April survey, appealed to the public and health professionals for more evidence about age discrimination in the health service. Over 1,000 people responded. Today's report, based on a close analysis of 150 cases, portrays a stark picture of systemic ageism within the NHS. It sets out the barriers which people over 50 face obtaining treatment, the less caring attitudes of health staff, and the way the fear of retaliation restricts complaints.

> **Prejudice** is an attitude that develops towards a particular group that has been identified in a negative way.
> **Stereotypes** develop from a simplified image of a group.

This can be reinforced through television and the media, so that, unless you have personal experience of older people, when you care for an older person you may shout at them (they are deaf) and suggest activities for them to do such as playing musical chairs (they act like children).

People may discriminate without realising it, but as care workers we must be careful not to use stereotypes when supporting patients and clients. At the same time, we need to be aware that everyone is an individual and we are not effective care workers if we treat everyone the same.

Discriminatory behaviour can include:

▶ racist and sexist jokes

▶ isolating clients with a mental health problem

▶ avoiding looking after someone who is from a different ethnic background from your own

▶ ignoring the needs of someone with HIV

▶ excluding certain residents from activities.

Discriminatory behaviour can also be indicated through:

▶ tone of voice (loud and aggressive)

▶ body language (distant and threatening)

▶ eye gaze (avoiding eye contact, or glaring).

## CASE STUDY ONE: JOHN

John has a learning disability and lives in a hostel with nine other men in their twenties who also have learning disabilities. There is a smoking policy in the house. Smoking is allowed in one area downstairs. John says he wants to smoke upstairs in his room. The staff are concerned about the fire risk as, two months earlier, John went to sleep with a lighted cigarette in his mouth, but the care assistant discovered him before any damage was done. John feels he is being treated unfairly because he has a learning disability.

## CASE STUDY TWO: MARIA

In a residential home in East London, all the residents are white men and women in their seventies. The care assistants include Maria, who is Afro-Caribbean. Mrs Bryant says, 'I don't want a darkie looking after me'.

What should the home manager do in these two situations?

Most health and social care organisations have an equal opportunities policy.

If you go on work experience try to look at the equal opportunities policy at the placement.

Although it is important to respect the values of clients and patients, you also need to be aware of the rights of other clients and service users, and of safety issues.

In order to promote anti-discriminatory practice, health and care organisations should:

▶ develop policies

▶ implement the policies

▶ give staff training in promoting better care to all clients

▶ have a complaints procedure so that patients and clients can seek redress.

All care workers find they like some of their patients more than others. This is natural. What you need to ask yourself is why you do not like a client? If it is because you feel awkward dealing with them because you do not understand their religion or culture, finding out about their views may be beneficial.

## Maintaining the confidentiality of information

Confidentiality is about keeping information private when it should be kept private. Think about the last time you went to see your doctor or practice nurse. What information would you be happy to give? What information would you feel uncomfortable about giving? How would you feel if your personal details were freely available to everyone?

A health and social care worker will know a great deal about the person they are looking after. It is essential that the information is kept confidential and not passed on without the client's permission.

Some information may have to be passed on from one care worker to another, or from a nurse to a doctor, but this must be done with the patient's permission.

The death of a patient does not give you the right to break confidentiality.

Clause 10 of the Code of Professional Conduct for nurses states that:

*'As a registered nurse, midwife or health visitor, you are personally account-able for your practice, and you must ... protect all confidential information about patients and clients obtained in the course of professional practice and make disclosures only with consent, where required by the order of a court or where you can justify disclosure in the wider public interest'* (UKCC)

Confidentiality can only be broken in exceptional circumstances. Every health and caring organisation will have a policy on confidentiality and the disclosure of information. Patients and clients have a right to know that their personal details are kept private and confidential. If you, as the care worker, need to disclose information this should be done:

▶ with the consent of the client or patient

▶ without the consent of the client or patient if required by law

▶ without the consent of the client or patient if the disclosure is seen to be in the public interest.

## CASE STUDY ONE:

You are on night duty on the children's ward. One of the children tells you her step-father is abusing her. What do you do?

## CASE STUDY TWO:

You are working on a male medical ward. A young man is brought in as an emergency. He has a bag with him that he asks you to keep in a safe place. He tells you that he has just arrived from India, and he is taking Schedule A drugs to his brother. He asks you to keep his secret.

In both these examples the duty of the nurse is quite clear, as in both cases it is a matter of public interest, but a lot of cases are quite difficult, and you would need to discuss them with your manager. In the two examples given, you would first report the matter to your line manager.

## Written records

Medical records are also covered by the same principles of confidentiality. There are usually procedures for keeping records safe in locked filing cabinets.

The 1987 *Access to Personal Files Act* allows patients to see their personal medical or social service files from this date. Notice to view your records is required. Doctors charge a fee for this service, and any record that may be damaging to the patient (in the opinion of the doctor) can be withheld. People with mental health problems could come into this category.

## Computer-based records

Many hospitals and surgeries now keep records on computer. *The Data Protection Act* (1984) covers all information that is held about people on computers. Every organisation that holds computer-based records must be registered, and there are guidelines for good practice that have to be followed.

1. The information must have been obtained legally and without deceit.

2. The information should only be used for the purpose for which it was collected.

3. The information should not be disclosed to anyone who has no right to see it.

4. There should be a proper security system, with a password required for access.

## Giving and receiving information on the telephone

With all phone calls dealing with personal information of patients and clients, care workers need to follow certain rules:

▶ make sure the person asking for information has a right to know

▶ refer anything you are unsure about to your manager

▶ if taking a message related to personal details, make sure that the message is recorded correctly, and pass the message on quickly, ensuring that only the person who needs to know sees it.

**CASE STUDY THREE: SARAH**

Sarah works in a rehabilitation unit which has computerised records for all the patients. Sarah is updating the records on screen at the duty desk. A relative wants to speak to her about one of the patients. The details on the screen are clearly visible. What should Sarah do?

GP practices have policies, especially related to giving information about test results. This is an example of one practice:

▶ if a patient phones about a result the receptionist will ask the person for their date of birth and address

▶ the receptionist will then ask the patient what kind of test it was

▶ if the receptionist is satisfied that he or she is speaking to the correct person they will give the information if the test is normal, or ask the patient to make an appointment with the doctor.

In most practices, if the results are abnormal the patient will be asked to make an appointment with the doctor. In many practices patients are asked to make another appointment to be told the results. This is especially important with results that patients may be worried about, such as pregnancy or the results of scans.

### Future developments

With new technology, the NHS is developing a lifelong electronic medical record of each patient, which can be accessed by GPs and hospitals. Some patients' groups are concerned about confidentiality. Certain information will not be available to other professionals without the patient's consent. This includes information about:

▶ patients with HIV and AIDs

▶ patients who are on fertility treatment

▶ patients who have been treated for sexually transmitted diseases.

## Promoting and supporting individual's rights to dignity, independence, health and safety

What do we mean by the term **rights**? Think for a moment what you understand to be your rights.

▶ Rights can be covered by laws, e.g. the right to drive a car at 17, the right to vote, or get married.

▶ Rights can also been seen as natural or as universal rights, e.g. the right to work, the right to have children, the right to make choices about what you do in your daily life.

In health and social care the rights of clients and patients are often stated in policies.

Figure 2.44 is an example of part of a Charter of Rights for older people in residential care. Most residential homes have a similar charter.

Figure 2.44 *An example of a Charter of Rights*

## CHARTER of RIGHTS

*As a resident of this Home you should enjoy the following rights:*

**Your Room**
- To have privacy by locking your room door and any cupboards inside your room.
- To have access to your own room when you wish.
- To entertain visitors in your room and to invite people to visit you whenever you wish. If you share a room, it is customary to ask the other occupant.

**The Home**
- To choose how you spend your day and who you spend your day with. You may wish simply to be alone.
- To eat when you wish during specified meal times.
- To select your meals from a choice on the menu.
- To assist in preparing the Home's menu.
- To use the Home's facilities for preparing snacks and beverages.
- To choose your bathing and washing times and who, if anyone, gives you support.
- To rise and go to bed when you please.
- To take part in any social and recreational activites that are organised.
- To contribute to the running of the Home by attending residents' committee meetings.
- To have influence over the spending of the Home's Amenity Fund through majority voting with other residents.
- To use the pay phone at any time for your private use.

You can find out about the rights of clients by looking at:

- codes of practice
- staff policies
- charters and other policies for service users
- standards of care.

## Codes of practice

There are many examples of codes of practice. Codes of conduct for social workers are currently being reviewed. Draft guidelines state that:

**Social workers must, to the best of their ability**:

- safeguard and promote the interests of service users and carers
- strive to maintain the trust and confidence of service users and carers

- respect the independence of service users and protect them as far as possible from danger or harm
- balance the rights of service users and carers with the 'interests of society'
- take responsibility for their own practice and learning
- justify public trust and confidence in social care services.

(*Source*: The General Social Care Council in England, the Northern Ireland Social Care Council, the Care Council for Wales, the Scottish Social Services Council.)

## Policies for staff

Nowadays most organisations have a range of policies. These can include:

- health and safety
- equal opportunities
- confidentiality
- complaints policies and procedures.

These policies give guidelines to staff, but also indicate how patients' and clients' rights should be protected.

If you go on work experience try to find some examples of policies.

## Charters for service users

### The Patients' Charter

The Patients' Charter was developed by the NHS in 1995. It is currently being revised, so that certain standards will be set nationally and other standards will be set locally, in order to take account of regional variations.

The Charter defines two terms:

1. **Rights** – these are what all patients will receive all the time.

2. **Expectations** – these are standards of service that the NHS is aiming to achieve. Sometimes these standards cannot be met for exceptional reasons (e.g. a flu epidemic).

According to the Patients' Charter, as a patient you have the right to:

- receive health care on the basis of clinical need, not on the ability to pay
- be registered with a GP and be able to change to another GP easily and quickly if you want to

▶ get emergency treatment at any time through your GP, the emergency ambulance service and hospital Accident and Emergency departments

▶ be referred to a consultant acceptable to you, when your GP thinks it is necessary, and be referred for a second opinion if you and your GP agree this is desirable.

**When you register with your GP** you have a right:

▶ to be offered a health check when you join a practice for the first time

▶ to ask for a health check-up if you are between 16 and 74 and have not seen the GP for the last three years

▶ be offered a health check in the GPs surgery, or at your own home if you prefer, if you are 75 or over.

## Standards of care

Local authorities have contracts with voluntary and other independent organisations, and as part of the service agreement the organisation has to provide care that reaches a certain standard. Social services also produce **standards of service statements** that tell clients what service they can expect.

Figure 2.45 shows an example of a Standards of Service Statement related to the assessment of children in need. Clients would be

---

**Figure 2.45** *A Standards of Service Statement*

### Our Standards:

● when you first contact us, we aim to let you know within one working day if you are eligible for an assessment

● we aim to complete your initial assessment within 7 working days of your first contact with us

● we aim to complete your core assessment within 42 working days of your first contact with us

● we will listen to the views of parents, young people and children, and record these

● we will contact other professionals dealing with your case (e.g. health, education)

● we will set a date to review any services we provide for you

● you will have a named contact person

● you will receive a copy of your assessment and care plan within 7 working days of their completion

*Source*: London Borough of Sutton

---

able to make a complaint if the service they received did not meet the standards in the statement.

**The client has rights to dignity**. When inspectors visit a home, they often use a checklist similar to Figure 2.46. If the rights of residents to dignity are respected:

▶ staff will knock on the door before entering (and wait for an answer)

▶ staff will address clients by the name they choose

▶ the privacy of the client will be respected

▶ the client will not be asked to do anything that is embarrassing and does not show respect to the individual.

> **Figure 2.46** *Checklist used when visiting a care home*

## A quality checklist

*Please tick the box which applies to the home in which you work.*

| | | |
|---|---|---|
| Do residents have their own private room? | Yes ☐ | No ☐ |

*If the answer to the above is no:*

| | | |
|---|---|---|
| Do all residents have personal lockable storage space? | Yes ☐ | No ☐ |
| Do residents have their own room key? | Yes ☐ | No ☐ |
| Do residents have their own front door key? | Yes ☐ | No ☐ |
| Are all the toilets lockable? | Yes ☐ | No ☐ |
| Can residents see visitors in their rooms or in a separate private meeting area? | Yes ☐ | No ☐ |
| Can residents eat in private if they wish? | Yes ☐ | No ☐ |
| Are there facilities for residents to continue old hobbies or take up new ones? | Yes ☐ | No ☐ |
| Can male and female residents mix freely in public and private areas? | Yes ☐ | No ☐ |
| Can residents cook a snack for themselves or make a drink? | Yes ☐ | No ☐ |
| Can residents choose when to go to bed? | Yes ☐ | No ☐ |
| Can residents choose when to get up? | Yes ☐ | No ☐ |
| Do all residents have a key worker? | Yes ☐ | No ☐ |
| Can residents arrange to eat at a different time? | Yes ☐ | No ☐ |

## CASE STUDY FOUR: MAVIS and MR NEWBOLD

Mr Newbold is a resident who has newly arrived at The Cedars residential home.

Before he retired he was headteacher at a well known boys school. Mr Newbold is sometimes rather forgetful. He enjoys reading the *Daily Telegraph* each day.

It is 8 am and Mr Newbold is resting in his room.

The door bursts open and Mavis, the care assistant appears.

*Mavis*: Ooh, love, I've had such a morning. I would have got to you sooner but we are short-staffed today, and then Mrs Brown on the landing had a 'little accident'. She didn't get to the loo in time and I had to clean her up. Oh well, we'd better get you ready for the bath. You do want a bath don't you?

*Mr N*: Oh dear, I don't really feel like it today.

*Mavis*: Well I'm running the bath now, so we'd better undress you and get you in.

*Mr N*: (struggling up and trying to undress ) Oh dear.

*Mavis*: Come on then, I have got the others to do still. Shall I help you? (grabs Mr Newbold and starts undressing him) Come on love, I haven't got all day.

# Activity

What do you think about Mavis and Mr Newbold?

Answer the following questions.

1. Is Mavis respecting the dignity of Mr Newbold?
2. Is she giving him a choice whether or not he has a bath?
3. Do you think Mr Newbold likes to be called *love* by someone he doesn't know?
4. How would you feel if you were Mr Newbold?
5. Why might Mavis behave the way she does?
6. What might be done to support Mr Newbold?

## Discussion

One of the first things you should have noticed, is how Mavis is discussing another client with Mr Newbold. This will make Mr Newbold wonder if Mavis discusses **him** with other residents. This is against principles of confidentiality.

Opening doors without knocking first shows a lack of respect for a person. Mavis speaks to Mr Newbold as if he is a child, and does not ask him how he wants to be addressed. Mavis could have offered a choice of a wash instead of a bath, which can be a struggle for an older person.

Perhaps Mavis does not realise what she is doing wrong; perhaps all the care workers behave in the same way in the home, which would mean that staff training is needed. Shortage of staff may mean that not enough staff are employed in the home and this can be stressful for everyone.

Gender issues can also be important. In some homes there are policies about male carers undertaking personal care for male clients. Mr Newbold could feel very embarrassed about a female carer rushing to undress him!

## Independence

Clients and patients should be supported so that they can be as independent as possible. Independence is linked to:

▶ self-respect

▶ responsibility

▶ being able to choose

▶ being an individual.

When we are babies and young children we are dependent on other people, but when we grow up we become independent individuals, with our own ideas, interests, friends and personal skills.

If we become:

▶ patients in hospital

▶ physically disabled

▶ mentally ill

▶ older

we are still the same individual.

People who are born with either learning or physical disabilities are also individuals who should be encouraged to be as independent as possible.

The word **care** should mean supporting someone to develop their full potential, but often it seems to mean controlling someone.

Promoting independence can involve risk. What risks would you need to consider if you were supporting someone like Claire?

## CASE STUDY ONE: CLAIRE

Claire is 45. She has been diagnosed with a serious mental illness (schizophrenia). She lives in a small residential home for six clients. After careful assessment of Claire's needs and abilities, the staff have encouraged Claire to go shopping and visit the cinema, be responsible for certain jobs in the home and make her own clothes.

Claire tells her visitors. 'I really like living here. The staff give me a lot of freedom. As long as I let them know, I can go out when I like. I went to the local pantomime with Bob (another resident) recently. The manager took us, but we came home on our own. I go to the town and buy material for the clothes I make myself. I sew them by hand in the dining room, when it isn't being used. I keep my room clean and do my own laundry.

I make tea for any visitors to the home. I like walking – I have bought some strong shoes as I walk a lot. I like to smoke and I can use a separate room for this.'

In some residential homes for all age groups, residents are encouraged to go out shopping, to the pub, to the local church, etc. Depending upon the condition of the client, each activity could have a risk attached, and it is important that the care worker discusses risks with the client and their relatives, and a decision is made as to whether the level of risk is acceptable. People who live in their own homes and want to maintain their independence may need to discuss issues of risk with their care worker.

We all take risks in our everyday life. Good care work is about supporting clients and patients to retain their independence and make choices about their lives.

Some client groups may not be able to ask for what they want, or have difficulty expressing their views. In order to ensure that the rights of these clients are fully supported, advocacy is used.

## Advocacy

Advocacy is when someone speaks on behalf of someone else who is unable to voice their views because of learning disabilities, mental health problems or for other reasons. The advocate can be a professional, a volunteer or a relative. The advocacy movement developed in the 1980s when many of the large institutions closed and people were moved into the community. Because these people had become institutionalised and were unable to communicate their needs effectively, advocates worked on their behalf.

Advocates can be volunteers who have used the service themselves (in the case of mental health service users). These are called **peer advocates**.

Skills needed by an advocate include:

▶ honesty, sensitivity and discretion

▶ patience and perseverance

▶ commitment to assisting service users

▶ good communication skills

▶ the ability to maintain confidentiality

▶ the ability to be supportive to the client.

People need advocacy in certain situations, such as:

▶ admission to and discharge from hospital

▶ community care assessments

▶ care management arrangements (e.g. review of care plan)

▶ changes in treatment

▶ requests to see medical records

▶ complaints

▶ requests to change doctors

▶ important visits to GPs

▶ access to education and work.

Apart from advocacy, where someone works on the behalf of the service user, there is also the development of self-advocacy, where clients are supported and helped so that they can speak out for themselves.

**Empowerment** – this term means the way in which a care worker encourages a client to take control of their own life. The client is also supported so that they can take an active part in deciding how their needs can be met.

## Health and safety

Health and safety is an important aspect in the hospital, residential home, day centre, or in the client's own home.

Figure 2.47 Health and safety checklist

| Risk Assessment | | Date initial assessment undertaken | |
|---|---|---|---|
| | | Assessment review date | |
| | | Signed | |
| **SAFE MOVEMENT** | | **Comments** | **Action required** |
| Are doorways, hall, stairs, landings and bedside areas well lit and free from clutter? | YES/NO | | |
| Do doors and windows in all rooms (especially the bathroom) open and shut easily? | YES/NO | | |
| Are any floor, stairs, steps, outside paths and all floor coverings damaged, uneven or slippery? | YES/NO | | |
| Are all areas free from trailing flexes? | YES/NO | | |
| Are firmly fitted handrails in use on both sides of the stairs, by toilet and bath? | YES/NO | | |
| **REACHING** | | | |
| Are shelves and cupboards in daily use in easy reach? | YES/NO | | |
| Are heavy items stored on high shelves or on top of wardrobes? | YES/NO | | |
| Can door butts, window catches, light switches, gas supply taps and post and milk deliveries be reached without difficult reaching and stooping? | YES/NO | | |
| **HEATING** | | | |
| Are all fires and heaters adequately guarded and well clear of furniture, curtains and bedclothes? | YES/NO | | |
| Are gas taps loose or are makeshift devices being used instead of proper gas connections? | YES/NO | | |
| Are all rooms well ventilated? | YES/NO | | |
| Are living rooms in daily use and bedrooms kept comfortably warm? | YES/NO | | |

Figure 2.47 is a checklist used in residential homes to assess health and safety. You could use this yourself at your work experience placement. As a care worker you have a responsibility for the health and safety of yourself and of your patients and clients. Many accidents happen in the home, both to older people and to young children.

## Activity

In your groups make a list of how you could make the following areas safer for:

1. older people
2. babies and young children
   - the kitchen
   - the bathroom
   - the hall and stairs and landing
   - the living room and bedroom
   - the garden.

Older people should be encouraged to keep active so that their mobility and balance is retained. Exercise classes have been set up in some areas; physiotherapists have visited people in their own homes and devised programmes for them to follow.

For more active older people, regular exercise such as yoga, dancing and walking can help prevent falls. In residential homes, exercise classes have been organised.

Well lit areas in the home, well fitting carpets and non-slip surfaces will guard against accidents. Bathmats and bathrails will protect against falls in the bathroom.

Kitchen utensils should be kept in accessible cupboards so that the person does not have to climb on a chair to reach them.

Help the Aged and Age Concern have produced useful leaflets. See if you can find some of them.

### Babies and young children

Accidents are the single largest cause of death in babies over one year. During the first 18 months of life, babies are unable to understand the idea of danger. These are some of the ways that babies can harm themselves:

- choking and suffocation
- burns and scalds
- falls
- poisoning
- cuts

- drowning
- electric shocks.

These are some of the things you might have mentioned in the section on the activity of babies and young children:

- not leaving the baby alone in the bath; making sure the water in the bath is not too hot
- using a stair gate, and perhaps bars on the windows, or making sure the windows fasten securely
- making sure all medicines are kept out of reach and in a locked cupboard
- making sure bleach and other household items that could be potentially dangerous are kept out of sight
- no hanging cords, from blinds for example, that could get caught round the baby's neck
- no small items left around that the baby could put in his/her mouth and choke on (parts of toys, nuts, etc)
- keeping all plastic bags away from babies and teaching young children not to put plastic bags on their heads
- never leaving a boiling pan unattended on the stove
- using a stair gate to keep the baby out of the kitchen
- keeping matches and lighters out of reach
- filling in or covering garden ponds.

RoSPA (the Royal Society for the Prevention of Accidents) provides information and advice on Safety in the Home. Their address is: Edgbaston Park, 353, Bristol Road, Birmingham B5 7ST.

Health and safety is a key concern for health and care workers, and we all need to do our best to reduce the number of accidents that occur each year in the home and elsewhere.

## Acknowledging an individual's personal beliefs and identity

People's values, beliefs and religion are part of their identity. Religious beliefs should be respected. The care worker can support the individual by:

- observing any dietary or other requirements
- respecting the wishes of the patient, for example by contacting the priest or minister if the patient requests it.

In some cases, the treatment of the patient may include therapy that is not allowed by the person's religion, so this must be discussed with the client and their wishes respected.

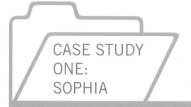

**CASE STUDY ONE: SOPHIA**

Sophia has just had her first baby. It was a difficult birth, and Sophia lost a great deal of blood. The consultant wanted to give Sophia a blood transfusion, but Sophia is a Jehovah's Witness and this religion bans the use of blood transfusions. The consultant could apply to the High Court to overrule Sophia's wishes. The risks to Sophia are explained to her and her husband and they remain adamant that they do not want a transfusion.

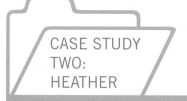

**CASE STUDY TWO: HEATHER**

Heather is four months pregnant with her first baby. When she has a scan, the doctor realises the baby has serious deformities. A second scan four weeks later confirms the original diagnosis. Heather is offered a termination. She is a committed Roman Catholic and will not consider a termination. The doctor arranges for her to see a neonatal specialist, who discusses the level of disability with her. Heather continues with her pregnancy.

In both these situations, the role of the health and care worker is to give Heather and Sophia information about possible outcomes, so that they are making an informed decision, and to support them after they have made that decision. The care worker should not pass judgments or make critical comments on the decisions made by clients and patients.

## Protecting individuals from abuse

For the GCSE, you need to be aware of the following:

- the definitions of abuse
- the individuals who may be at risk
- how the law relates to abuse.

## What is abuse?

Abuse can be defined as deliberate and intended harm to another person, or a way of treating them so as to cause harm.

Health and care workers often care for people who are vulnerable to abuse. This abuse can be:

- **Physical** – punching, kicking, slapping or restraining people. It could also include handling people roughly, when assisting with bathing, moving clients, or toileting.
- **Sexual** – sexual exploitation of a child or other person. This could include touching and other acts against the person without their consent.
- **Psychological** – humiliating or harassing a client, bullying and shouting at someone.
- **Financial** – theft of money or possessions, or fraud. Putting pressure on a client to leave them money in their will or to give them money. Keeping control of someone's money.
- **Neglect** – deprivation of food, warmth, comfort or medical assistance.

### Individuals who are likely to be at risk:

- children
- people with mental health problems
- people with learning disabilities
- people with physical disabilities
- older people.

### Individuals who may abuse:

- parents and other relatives
- care workers and other professionals
- other children/clients.

### Where may abuse take place?

- In the person's own home
- At school
- In a formal care setting
- In other settings, such as outings, camps, leisure centres, etc.

## CASE STUDY ONE: NORMAN

Norman is 75. He has Alzheimer's Disease. He is a patient in a long stay unit for patients with dementia. Because of his condition, it is difficult to communicate with him. He spends the day in the living room of the unit. There are 26 patients in the unit with dementia, and there are only three staff on duty. Norman is in a special chair, but he keeps rolling out of it and falling on to the floor. The nurses are concerned that he will fall and hurt himself, so they decide to tie him into the chair.

What is the problem here? What are Norman's rights?

Many organisations have a restraint policy, which indicates when it is acceptable to secure a client so they cannot harm themselves or others. It is important that staff follow the guidelines.

Is this an example of physical abuse?

## CASE STUDY TWO: DAVID

David Smith's niece, Susan, decided she wanted him to come and live with her and her husband Mike. The social worker Mary visited the flat, where there was a room for David. As time went by, the social worker became increasingly anxious about David. He was often in bed when she came in the afternoon, and sometimes there was no reply to her knock on the door, although she was sure there was someone in the house. Mike had lost his job and money was tight. The winter was cold and Mary decided to see the family as there had been no response to phone calls and letters. When she finally visited, she saw David in his room. The room was very cold, without any heating. The room smelt of urine and excrement. David had a bad cough. The GP was called and David was admitted to hospital, where he later died of pneumonia. When doctors examined David they found he was undernourished and covered in bruises. The inquest found that he had died of neglect. In the inquiry that followed, it was found that the only reason Susan and Mike wanted to have David in their home was so that they would have access to his various allowances and benefits, including his bank account. Most of his possessions had been sold.

This case study shows that financial abuse can also lead to other forms of abuse. As increased numbers of vulnerable people live in the community, it is important that care workers are vigilant in protecting them from abuse.

## Children and abuse

There have been various cases reported in the media where children have been abused by their parents or carers and by workers in residential homes.

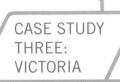

### CASE STUDY THREE: VICTORIA

In 2001, a Government inquiry was launched into the death of an eight-year-old girl, Victoria Climbie. Victoria had suffered 128 injuries, some inflicted with a bicycle chain, and had been repeatedly sexually abused. The child had come to England from Africa in 1999 to be looked after by her aunt and her boyfriend. Although social services had been alerted about the possible abuse Victoria was suffering, nothing was done to protect her. After spending the winter months tied up and left in a bath, she finally died of hypothermia (lowered body temperature) in February 2000. Victoria's aunt and boyfriend were found guilty of child cruelty and murder and were jailed for life.

## How can we protect individuals from abuse?

▶ By raising awareness of possible problems.

▶ By noting and recording any signs of possible abuse. These could include:

  ▸ **physical signs**, such as bruising, burns, scalds, injuries (including fractures), AND/OR

  ▸ **emotional signs**, such as changes in behaviour, including sleep patterns, bedwetting, appearing tense or frightened, changes in eating patterns, depression.

▶ By reporting incidents to the appropriate organisation.

▶ By training staff so they are aware of the procedures to follow.

### How does the Law relate to abuse?

The *Children Act* (1989) requires social services to provide protection from abuse for all children in their area. This has been additionally reinforced through the *Modernising Social Services Programme* (1998) which has tightened up policies related to children's services, especially with the development of a register for all people who work with children. Social services are also required to maintain an up to date register of people working with children.

## Providing individualised care

Care programmes are ways of providing individualised care through a care plan.

Before developing a care plan a care worker needs to:

▶ identify a client's needs and values

▶ gain information from the client, carer and other people who may be significant (e.g. medical staff).

### Individual care plans

Care plans state what will be provided for a client, by whom, when, where and how. Care plans are drawn up with the carer, service user and the care worker. Care plans cover what the client has a right to expect. Care plans are reviewed at set times, as the care needed may change, and the care plan should be updated to reflect any changes. Figure 2.48 shows an example of a care plan.

Care plans are important written records and may be used in court, so they must be legible, clearly stated, signed and dated by the care worker.

Figure 2.49 is part of an assessment document and shows how the individual needs of a client are assessed.

Look at the following case study and identify Mary's needs.

The care planning cycle is a continuous process and the care plan needs to be continuously reviewed as people's needs change over a period of time.

▶ Their needs may reduce, for example if they are attending a physiotherapy or rehabilitation programme.

▶ Their needs may increase, for example if their physical or mental health gets worse.

CASE STUDY
THREE:
MARY

Mary is 36. She has cerebral palsy and uses a wheelchair to get about. She has a son of five and a daughter of seven. Her husband is her main carer. She uses the local dial-a-ride service when she needs transport to the clinic. The family live in a ground floor flat, and there is a shower that Mary can use. Mary's speech is slow. She has difficulty holding a knife, spoon or fork. Apart from going to the clinic by the transport service she cannot get out. Because she sits for long periods in the chair she can get uncomfortable. She has a catheter in place to remove urine, and this is changed by the district nurse.

Figure 2.48 *Example of a care plan*

| CARE PLAN | | | | Name | Mrs Brown. aged 80 | |
|---|---|---|---|---|---|---|
| Date | No. | Needs/Problems | Rational/Aims | Action | Signature | Date Completed & Signature |
| 16/1/02 | 1 | Diabetes control | To stabilise diabetes | To refer to G.P. for assessment | DN | |
| | 2 | Hearing difficulty | To improve hearing | To refer to Audiology Dept. | DN | |
| | 3 | Problems of moving | To improve mobility | To refer to occupational therapist | | |
| | | round house | and safety | | DN | |
| | | | | | | |
| 16/2/02 | 1 | Diabetes | To stabilise diabetes | Blood to be taken by nurse each week | DN | DN 16/2/02 |
| | | | | and urine to be tested by Mrs Brown each day. | | |
| | 2 | Hearing | To improve hearing | Still awaiting appointment | DN | |
| | 3 | Problems of mobility | To improve mobility | Rails put up in hallway | | OT 16/2/02 |
| | | | | Advice given on safety and excercise | | |
| | | | | | | |
| | | | | | | |
| | | | | | | |
| | | | | | | |

**Figure 2.49** *An example of an assessment document*

| Relevant nursing history _____ |
| --- |

**Relevant medical history** _____

**General observations** _____

| T | P | R | BP | | **Height** |
| --- | --- | --- | --- | --- | --- |

**Urine** _____ **Weight** _____

**Eyes** Glasses _____ Date last test _____

**Hearing** _____ Type of Aid _____

**Mouth Dentures** _____ **Fitting** _____

**Speech or language problems** _____

| Mobility – Can do | Alone | With help |
| --- | --- | --- |
| Stand | | |
| Pull to sitting | | |
| Roll over in bed | | |
| Walk | | |
| Stairs | | |
| Feed | | |
| Dress | | |
| Bath | | |
| Use toilet | | |
| Shopping | | |
| Cooking | | |
| Use public transport | | |

**Skin** _____

**Feet** _____ **Chiropody** _____

**Nutrition** _____ M on W _____

**Elimination** Bladder _____

**Bowels** _____

**Laundry service** _____ Disposal service _____

*Source*: SouthWest London Community Trust

## Assessment of needs

This can be a lengthy process. At the moment, dual assessments are being developed, where a joint assessment of a person's health and care needs and their financial position is done in a single process.

**Drawbacks of assessments done separately** by the health and care worker:

▶ the client gets confused about which care worker is responsible for which area of support

▶ lengthy process, with several people visiting the person to undertake assessment

▶ problems of communication between different key workers.

**Drawbacks of joint assessment:**

▶ can take a long time in one visit and be very tiring for the client

▶ nurses feel uncomfortable asking for financial details of patients

▶ staff training is needed.

In order to provide an individualised care service it is essential that the client, carer or other relative is closely involved with the care professional in developing a programme of care.

## Supporting individuals through alternative approaches to communication

Clients or care workers:

▶ can speak different languages

▶ can have hearing loss or limited vision.

Some client groups:

▶ may find it difficult to speak

▶ may have limited understanding.

We can see that there can be difficulties communicating with different groups, but if we are going to deliver care according to the principles of the value base, we need to be aware of how we can overcome these barriers.

### *Different languages*

**Mistakes** that are made:

▶ the health professional talks loudly to the patient, thinking this might help

▶ the health professional may try sign language which may add to the confusion.

**Communication barrier** due to **language problems** means that:

▶ the care worker becomes irritated and frustrated

▶ the patient does not understand what is going on and cannot contribute to the discussion of care or future planning.

CASE STUDY
ONE:
MIDWIVES

Midwives in West London discovered that very few Bangladeshi women were attending antenatal clinics, and this meant that sometimes problems with the pregnancy were not identified. A link worker scheme was set up. Bangladeshi women who had a good understanding of English were recruited and trained. In specialist areas such as midwifery, it is important that the **link worker** is able to act as interpreter between the doctor or midwife and the patient, but the link worker also needs to have insight into the difficulties that may be caused by the difference in culture. Asian women tend to look away from a professional person as an act of respect, but the doctor may interpret this non-verbal communication as hostility or lack of interest. The link worker can act as a bridge between the two cultures.

Possible solutions:

▶ use of interpreters in face to face situations – these can either be staff working in the home or hospital, or relatives

▶ use of leaflets and other written information in the patient's own language. The *Patients' Charter* is available in many languages, and many hospitals are providing information in languages other than English. It is difficult to cover all languages. In the London area alone, it is estimated that there are over 300 different languages.

▶ Use of **Language Line**. This is a specialist telephone service that interprets phone calls. It is used by NHS Direct.

### Hearing loss

In the UK approximately three in every 1000 children are born with a hearing loss. The majority of deaf children are born to hearing parents. The chance of having a hearing loss increases with age. It is estimated that one in five of all adults and more than half of all people over 60 have a hearing loss..

▶ At least 50,000 people are estimated to use BSL (British Sign language).

▶ At least 154,000 people lip read.

▶ 21,000 people are both deaf and blind.

Attempts are being made to facilitate communication with deaf people:

▶ in some hospitals and residential homes there may be an interpreter who can sign (using BSL) so that communication between the care worker /professional is maintained

▶ many local adult education centres run classes for people to learn BSL

▶ RNID (Royal National Institute for the Deaf) gives useful information on learning how to sign. Figure 2.50 shows the basic alphabet for signing. Lip-reading is very tiring for the person who is doing the lip-reading, so it is helpful if there is someone present who can use sign language.

Figure 2.51 is a useful way of remembering how to support people who lip-read. Research done by RNID in 1998 showed that visiting the doctor is very difficult for people who have a hearing problem. The most common problems were:

▶ doctors being unable to communicate effectively with patients

▶ lack of signing facilities

▶ making an appointment.

Can you think of possible solutions to these problems?

# Activity

Next time you are looking at a news programme on the television, turn the sound down and see how much you can understand. You will notice that your understanding is helped if there are prompts, such as pictures, which give you an idea about the subject.

Try the same activity with a friend who is mouthing words rather than saying them, and see how well you do.

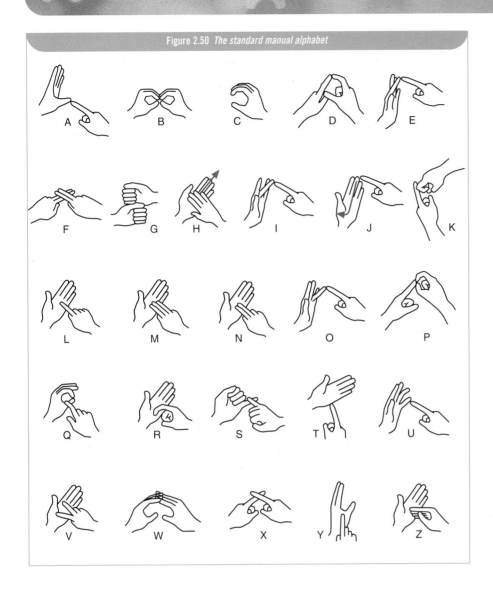

Figure 2.50 *The standard manual alphabet*

### Deaf blind

In the UK it is estimated that 21,000 people are deaf blind. Because communication is so difficult with this group of people, as they cannot see non-verbal communication as well as being unable to hear, touch is a very important source of communication.

There is an alphabet that can be used by a deaf blind person, but very often other communication movements can be used, similar to Makaton (see pages 183–184).

### Limited vision

Visual impairment can be due to a variety of causes.

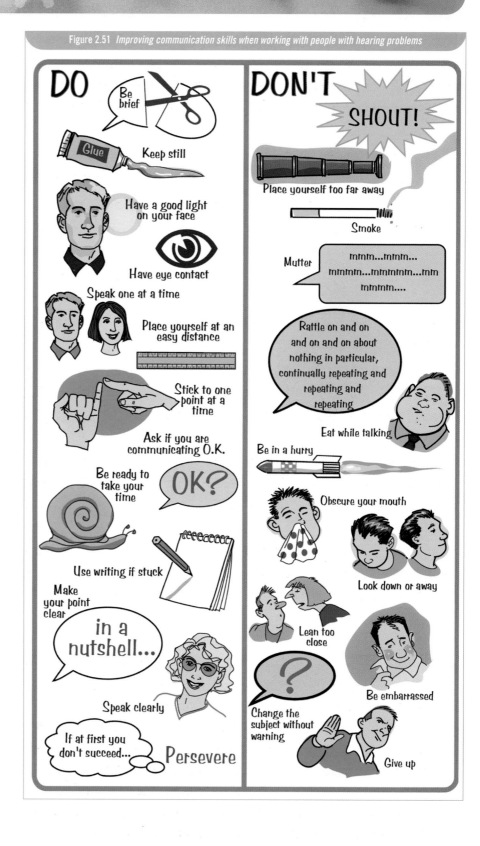

Figure 2.51 *Improving communication skills when working with people with hearing problems*

As a carer, you need to ask the visually impaired person what is the most helpful way for you to assist them. If you cannot see, it is quite frightening if someone rushes up to you and grabs you by the arm. It may be more helpful if the blind person takes the arm of the helper.

If you are working with a visually impaired person:

▶ introduce yourself – the person may not be aware of your presence

▶ sit or stand in the position that suits the blind person best

▶ reinforce your conversation with clear speech, and touch the person if appropriate

▶ don't grab the person – ask them if they need help to go somewhere and what help they need

▶ use tone of voice rather than facial expression to communicate mood and response

▶ do not rely on non-verbal communication

▶ make sure that information is transferred on to something that the person can hear, such as tapes, if braille is inappropriate or not possible.

Many blind people complain that much of the information about health and social care is in leaflets. Can you think of ways you could give information to blind people about the health services available to them?

If someone becomes visually impaired, for example, due to disease, the OT may visit the home and advise on ways of adapting cookers and other appliances so that the person's independence is maintained.

### Difficulty in speaking

There are several groups of people who have difficulty speaking. This could be due to problems from birth, such as cerebral palsy, or difficulties in later life due to accidents or strokes. According to the Stroke Association, every five minutes someone in England and Wales has a stroke. Ten thousand people each year have speech problems as a result of a stroke. The Stroke Association runs programmes for people who have **aphasia** (difficulty speaking). Speech and language therapists work with aphasic patients. The Stroke Association also produces visual aids (see Figure 2.52) that patients can use, so that they can communicate by pointing at the relevant picture.

Here are some **do's and don'ts** for when you are communicating with someone who has a speech difficulty.

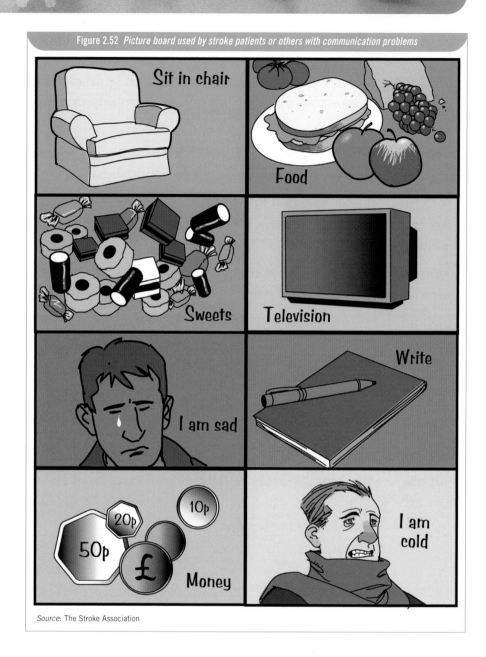

Figure 2.52 *Picture board used by stroke patients or others with communication problems*

*Source*: The Stroke Association

1. Do not finish the person's sentence for them.
2. Give them plenty of time.
3. If you are not clear what they have said, ask them to repeat it.
4. Use picture cards, computers or other communication means.
5. Do not forget that the person can still hear, even if they cannot speak clearly.

### Limited understanding

There are at least two client groups you may work with who have limited understanding.

1. **People with learning disabilities** – people with leaning disabilities can have different levels of understanding, so it is important that you identify the level, either by speaking to a care worker, or by talking to the person. It is important that you:

   ▶ talk to the person at the right level, using words they understand and check they understand you

   ▶ repeat things so that you make sure they understand you

   ▶ respond to questions they ask you at the right level

   ▶ remain patient, and be prepared to take time over communication

   ▶ support verbal communication with drawings and diagrams if and when appropriate.

---

### Makaton

Makaton is a language programme that has been developed for people with communication and learning difficulties. It was devised in 1972 by Margaret Walker, a speech therapist. It is used in the UK in pre-school settings, and in schools, day centres, hospitals and clinics, and in the homes of people with severe communication and learning difficulties. It has been adapted for use in 40 other countries. Many of the signs used in makaton are from BSL.

Makaton uses signs and facial expressions. Speech is always used with signs. Figure 2.53 shows some of the basic signs.

It is possible to learn Makaton at local education centres. Makaton has helped some groups to communicate effectively for the first time.

---

2. **Alzheimer's Disease and dementia**

   With dementia and Alzheimer's Disease, communication can be affected because the client can suffer from short-term memory loss, as well as confusion about time and place.

   If you visit a residential home for people with dementia you may find that the staff make every effort to encourage the clients to be aware of time and place.

   There may be a board showing the day of the week and the date. Photographs of recent events in the home may be displayed. Some activities may include **reminiscence therapy**, where photos and past events are discussed. An example of this would be a scrapbook of local events during World War II.

When talking to someone with dementia you need to **repeat information** as often as necessary. This is because of the problems of short-term memory loss, so you may be asked questions such as What time is it? What is for lunch today? Where are we going? Who are you? frequently, so it is important that you remain patient and repeat the information.

You also need to :

▶ keep conversation clear and simple

▶ use simple pictures or written information if this helps

▶ try to keep the patient in reality

▶ if the client says something strange, for instance if a 70-year-old says he is expecting to see his father that afternoon, do not assume he is confused but check the truth of the statement

▶ use distraction tactics if the client seems determined to do something dangerous to himself or others.

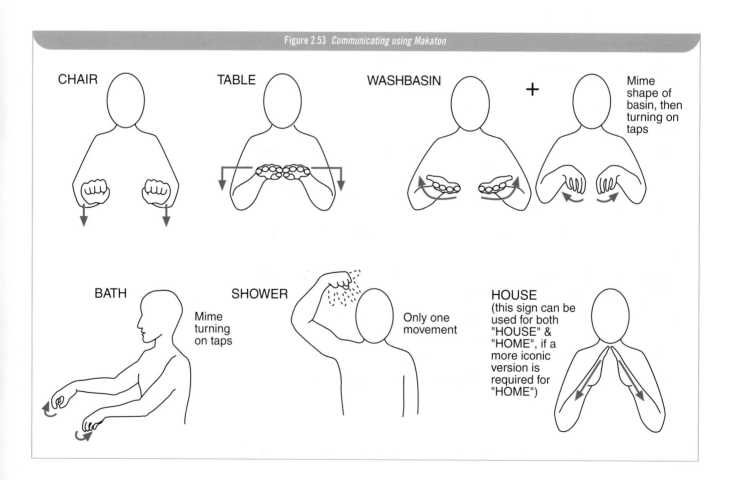

Figure 2.53 *Communicating using Makaton*

We have now seen how communication methods can be adapted so that clients and patients can be supported towards a more independent life.

# RESOURCES

## References used in this chapter

Asterisked references could also be useful resources for students.

Bell, L. (1999) *Care Fully. A Handbook for Home Care Assistants*. Age Concern*

Crabtree, H. and Warner, L. (1999) *Too much to take on. A Report on Young Carers and Bullying*. The Princess Royal Trust

*Just the Job. Care and Community* (1997) London, Hodder and Stoughton*

*Just the Job. Medicine and Health* (1997) London, Hodder and Stoughton*

*Just the Job. Nursing and Therapies* (1997) London, Hodder and Stoughton*

*Modernising Social Services* White Paper (1998) HMSO

*The New NHS, Modern, Dependable* (1997) DOH

Nolan, Y. (1998) Care. NVQ level 2*

Richards, J. (1999) *The Complete A–Z Health and Social Care Handbook*. London, Hodder and Stoughton*

*Social Trends* (1999) HMSO

*Social Trends* (2001) HMSO

Thomson, H. et al. (1997) *Health and Social Care for Advanced GNVQ*, Second Edition. London, Hodder and Stoughton

Thomson, H. et al. (2000) *Health and Social Care Intermediate GNVQ*, Second Edition. London, Hodder and Stoughton

Thomson, H. et al. (2000) *Health and Social Care. Vocational A level*, Third Edition. London, Hodder and Stoughton

Thomson, H. and Meggitt, C. (1997) *Human Growth and Development for Health and Social Care*. London. Hodder and Stoughton

Warner, I. and Wexler, S. (1998) *8 Hours a Day and Taken for Granted*. The Princess Royal Trust

*Wellards NHS Handbook 1999/2000* (1999) JMH Publishing

Worsley, J. (1998 ) *Taking Good Care. A handbook for care assistants*. Age Concern*

## Other resources

References that could be useful are marked with an asterisk in the section above.

Most local authorities and local voluntary groups provide a range of materials that are relevant to the course.

If you contact the head office of a national organisation, send a stamped addressed envelope and at least 60 pence in stamps to go towards the costs. You may find additional information on websites, and these are listed under the *useful addresses* section below.

The weekly publication *Community Care* has relevant articles. It also has a website address www.community-care.co.uk

Local free newspapers usually cover health issues and include examples of jobs in health and social care in the job advertisement section.

# Useful addresses

You may find it quicker to access information you need through the Internet. Many organisations now have their own websites, some of which are listed on page 188.

Barnardo's
Tanners Lane
Barkingside
Essex IGB IQG

Child Poverty Action Group
1–5 Bath Street
London ECU9 PY

NSPCC (National Society for the Prevention of Cruelty to Children)
National Centre
42 Curtain Road
London EC2A 3NH

Age Concern England
Astral House
1268 London Road
London SW16 4ER

Childline
Royal Mail Building
50 Studd Street
London N1 OQW

Winged Fellowship Trust (Holidays for People with Disabilities)
Angel House
20–32 Pentonville Road
London N1 9XD

Carers National Association
20/25 Glasshouse Yard
London EC1A 4JS

British Red Cross
9 Grosvenor Crescent
London SW1X 7EJ

RNIB (Royal National Institute for the Blind)
224 Great Portland Street
London W1W 5AA
www.rnib.org.uk

RNID (Royal National Institute for Deaf People)
19–23 Featherstone Street
London EC1 8SL
www.rnid.org.uk

The Stroke Association
CHSA House
123–127 Whitecross Street
London
EC1Y 8JJ

# Careers advice

Degree Programmes in Nursing
UCAS
Fulton House
Jessop Avenue
Cheltenham
Glos GL50 3SH

Health Service Careers
PO Box 204
London SE99 7UW
Tel. 0207 6366287
Provides leaflets on different careers in the Health Service

NHS Careers
Tel 0845 6060655 (24 hours)
Email. advice@nhscareers.nhs.uk

## Advice on careers in nursing or midwifery

NHS Careers
PO Box 376
Bristol BS99 3EY
Contact for advice on minimum requirements for entry into nursing

NMAS
Rosehill
New Barn Lane
Cheltenham
Glos GL52 3LZ
Tel. 01242 223707
For application package details for entry to nursing
Tel 01242 544949 for general enquiries

Professional Association of Nursery Nurses
2 St James Court
Friar Gate
Derby
DE1 1BT
Leaflets for nannies, setting up nurseries, etc.

## Useful websites

www.nhsdirect.nhs.uk NHS Direct Online for health information and guidance

www.patient.co.uk Patient information publications

www.nice.org.uk National Institute for Clinical Excellence

www.healthcentre.org.uk/hc/library/gp.htm useful links for patients and health-care professionals

www.hsj.co.uk Health Service Journal

www.nursingtimes.net Nursing Times

www.doh.gov.uk Department of Health

www.show.scot.nhs.uk The NHS in Scotland

www.dhssni.gov.uk Ths NHS in Northern Ireland

www.ons.gov.uk Office for National Statistics

www.doh.gov.uk/pointh.htm Department of Health publications on the Internet

www.nhs.uk/nhsplan The NHS Plan 2000

# Glossary

**adoption**
the legal transfer of an infant or child from the birth family to another family.

**advocacy**
in which someone speaks on the behalf of someone else, who is unable to voice their views because of learning disabilities, mental health problems or other reasons. The advocate can be a professional, volunteer or a relative.

**ageism**
discrimination based on age, which means that a person is treated unfairly or differently from others because of their age.

**alternative medicine (or therapy)**
treatment of different conditions that focuses on the whole person (**holistic**) rather than just concentrating on the disease itself.

**assessment**
formal method of identifying the health and social needs of a service user in order to set up a care plan.

**Benefits Agency**
the agency within the Department of Social Security which is responsible for the assessment and payment of social security benefits.

**care plan**
the plan of treatment and care decided upon jointly by the service user and the named nurse or key worker.

**carer**
person who takes on the responsibility for the care and support of a person who cannot fully support themselves.

**case conference**
formal meeting of professionals, service users, carers and family to plan future action.

**charities**
non-profit making organisations set up to support different groups.

**Child Health Surveillance Programme**
system of development checks carried out in the first eight years of life.

**chiropody**
treatment of feet, also known as **podiatry**.

**chiropractic**
alternative therapy involving manipulation of the spine.

**clinician**
any health professional who is directly involved in the treatment and care of patients (e.g. midwife, doctor).

**code of conduct**
professional code of behaviour and practice drawn up by a professional body to set standards (e.g. UKCC).

**district nurse**
qualified nurse who works closely with the GPs and is employed by the Community Trust.

**domiciliary services**
health and social care services that take place in the service user's home.

**foster care**
care of child or children by the local authority in a family group. This can be provided by foster carers paid by the LA, or by a fostering agency.

**geriatrician**
doctor who specialises in the diseases and disorders of older people.

**health authorities**
regional and district – bodies that identify the medical needs of an area and manage the administration and development of health services.

**health improvement programme (HImP)**
national, regional and local plans to improve the health of the population, focusing on particular needs relevant to the area.

**health visitor**
a registered nurse with additional training, who works in the community to advise and support children under the age of eight and their families. The role has recently been expanded to include health promotion, including continence advice.

**Home Care Services**
community team that provides social care for clients in their own homes.

**homeopathy**
alternative therapy using natural substances to help the body heal itself in a range of conditions, e.g. eczema.

**hospice**
usually a small unit set up to care for the dying (terminally ill).

**independent sector**
the group of agencies that provide health and social care independently from statutory providers. They can be private (profit making) or voluntary (non-profit making).

**informal care**
care (usually unpaid) that is given by friends, family or neighbours.

**key worker**
a named person who ensures that the care plan is followed and care is given to the client/patient. In health care, there would be a named nurse who is responsible for the care of certain patients.

**NHS Charter**
Charter outlining the standards of care, including waiting times, patients can expect from the NHS.

**NHS Direct**
a 24-hour phone service staffed by nurses.

**NHS Executive**
central management organisation in the NHS.

**NHS trusts**
hospitals or community services which are independent bodies and employ staff to deliver medical care.

**occcupational therapist (OT)**
therapist who treats patients in hospital and in the community and encourages independent living.

**optician**
professional trained to examine and test eyes and prescribe lenses.

**orthopaedic specialist**
surgeon specialising in the disease, injury and problems of bones and joints.

**osteopathy**
alternative treatment of muscles, bones and joints using massage, manipulation and other techniques.

**paediatrician**
qualified doctor who specialises in treating children.

**pharmacist**
qualified professional who dispenses prescriptions and gives advice to patients.

**physiotherapist**
professional who treats a range of conditions, including post-operative rehabilitation, using exercise, massage and other therapies.

**Primary Care Group (PCG)**
set up in 1999 to deliver primary health care and to develop links with the secondary sector (hospital services). They will develop to become **PCTs (trusts)**, when they will commission and provide services in health care.

**Primary Health Care Team (PHCT)**
includes GPs, nurses, pharmacists, opticians, and other health workers.

**risk assessment**
procedure that assesses the risks in the environment to the service user (e.g. unsafe home). It can also be applied to people with mental health problems when a doctor would decide whether the patient is a danger to himself or to others.

**secondary services**
medical care that is given in hospital rather than in the primary care setting.

**self advocacy**
the service user is encouraged and assisted to speak on their own behalf about the services they need.

**speech and language therapist**
professional trained to help adults and children overcome a range of problems related to speech and swallowing. Problems can include stammering, dysphagia (difficulty in swallowing) and aphasia (difficulty in speaking, for example after a stroke or head injury).

**tertiary care**
medical care offered at a specialist hospital, e.g. oncology (cancer), neurology (to do with the brain and spinal cord) or cardiac (heart).

# ANSWERS

**Use of the NHS**, page 83

1. Phone NHS Direct/see pharmacist

2. See the pharmacist

3. Dial 999

4. See the pharmacist or GP

5. Dial 999 or go to A & E

**Children's services**, page 99

1. Health visitor

2. Speech and language therapist

3. Enuresis clinic

4. Community dental clinic

5. Health visitor

6. Audiology service

7. Community paediatrician

8. Child Psychiatrist

9. Educational psychologist

**Carers**

Relationship to cared for, page 105

1. Spouse or partner

2. Parents in law or other

Age of carer, page 106

1. 17%

2. 65%

3. 34% are over 65 (figures do not add up to 100%)

**Direct/Indirect care**, page 121

▶ porter – indirect care

▶ health visitor – direct care

▶ practice manager – indirect care

▶ practice nurse – direct care

▶ chiropodist – direct care

# Promoting health and well-being | 3

## CHAPTER CONTENT

This chapter will help you learn about:

▶ definitions of health and well-being

▶ common factors that affect health and well-being and the different effects they can have on individuals and groups across the lifespan

▶ methods used to measure an individual's physical health

▶ ways of promoting and supporting health improvement for an individual or small group.

The knowledge that you gain will help you look after your own health and well-being and understand ways of promoting health and well-being for others.

## UNDERSTANDING HEALTH AND WELL-BEING

### Definitions of health and well-being

There are several different ways of thinking about health and well-being.

'At least I've still got my health.' When someone says this, what do they mean by **health**? It is likely that you understand their meaning, but it is difficult for you to define the word 'health'. Different people will have different ideas about health. There is a range of definitions of health and well-being used by ordinary people, professionals and different organisations.

## Activity

Before you read any further, think how *you* would define 'being healthy'. Ask a few of your friends what definition they would give.

# Activity

1. Look at the glossary at the end of the chapter to check the meaning of **illness**, **disease**, and **sickness**.

2. Think about occasions on which you have been unwell and decide whether these episodes would have been classed as illness, disease, or sickness.

There are three different definitions of health commonly given.

## 1. Negative definition of health and well-being

*'The absence of physical illness, disease and mental distress'.*

Many people only think about health when they are thinking about illness or health problems. This means they may give a negative definition of health, such as 'not being ill' or 'being free of pain'.

The medical definition of health is often thought to be 'absence of disease'. This is a negative definition. It does not describe health as a positive state. It views health as being when you are not classified as sick or in need of medical help. It ignores the fact that health is about feeling well, energetic and at ease. It may also mean that people with disabilities or **chronic conditions** (see glossary) may be labelled as 'sick' or 'diseased' when they are otherwise healthy.

## 2. Positive definition of health and well-being

*'The achievement and maintenance of physical fitness and mental stability.'*

Some people think more positively of health as fitness and well-being. They may associate health with moods and feelings, and a sense of balance.

## 3. Holistic definition of health and well-being

*'Health and well-being are the result of a combination of physical, social, intellectual and emotional factors.'*

A widely used definition of health came from the **World Health Organisation (WHO)** in 1948. This defines health as:

*'a state of complete physical, mental and social well-being and not merely the absence of disease or infirmity.'*

This has been widely quoted because it goes much further than just seeing health as freedom from disease. Instead, health is viewed as all-round well-being (Figure 3.1). However, it has been criticised for two main reasons.

1  It is seen as too idealistic. How often do you really feel yourself to be in a state of 'complete well-being'?

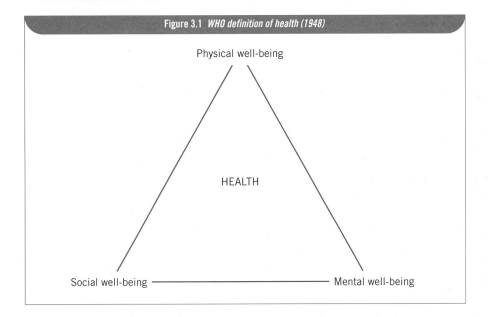

Figure 3.1 *WHO definition of health (1948)*

2 It does not consider the ability to adapt to the changes that we all face throughout life. In the light of these criticisms, a more recent WHO definition of health is:

*'The extent to which an individual or group is able, on the one hand, to realise aspirations and satisfy needs and, on the other hand, to change or cope with the environment. Health is a positive concept emphasising social and personal resources as well as physical capabilities.'*

This definition shows that:

▶ health is an important part of our everyday lives

▶ it is a positive concept

▶ health is a much wider concept than freedom from disease

▶ health takes into account the whole person

▶ health is related to our ability to cope and adapt to change

▶ health might be understood in different ways by different individuals and groups.

# Physical, intellectual, emotional and social health

The WHO definitions are **holistic** definitions as they encourage the view of health as concerned with the whole person and not just their physical state. When thinking about a person's health you should think about physical, intellectual, emotional and social aspects (Figure 3.2). You will be able to remember these if you think of the word 'PIES' (Figure 3.3).

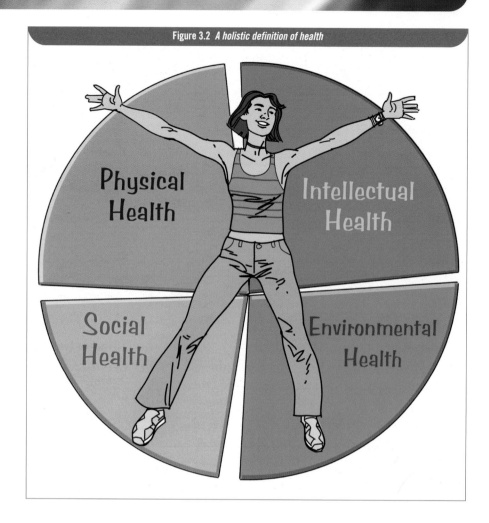

Figure 3.2 *A holistic definition of health*

- **Physical health** – this is concerned with the physical functioning of the body. Physical health is the easiest aspect of health to measure.

- **Intellectual health (or mental health)** – this is concerned with the ability to think clearly and rationally. It is closely linked to emotional and social health (see below).

- **Emotional health** – this is concerned with the ability to recognise emotions such as fear, joy, grief, frustration and anger, and to express such emotions appropriately. Emotional health also includes the ability to cope with anxiety, stress and depression.

- **Social health** – this is concerned with the ability to relate to others and to form relationships with other people.

You must remember that these different aspects of health are not separate but overlap and influence one another. For example, the pain and discomfort of an illness may make you unhappy. In this case, your physical health is influencing your emotional health.

Figure 3.3 *PIES – health is a combinaton of personal, intellectual, emotional and social development*

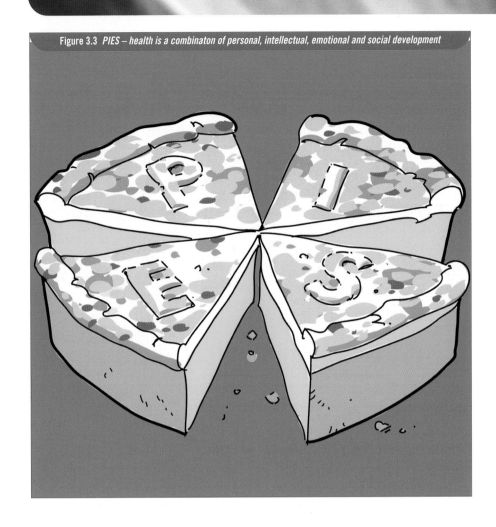

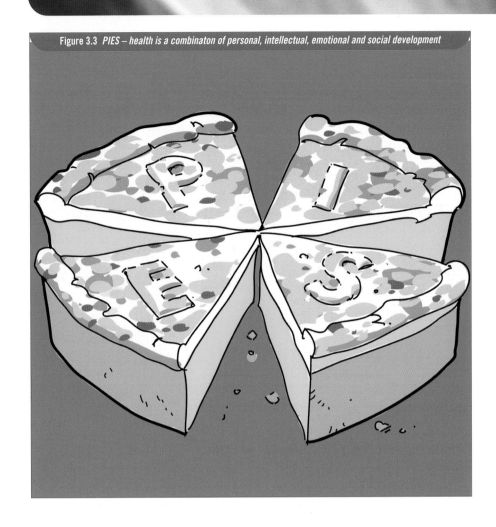

CASE STUDY
ONE:
SHAZIYA

Shaziya is a sixteen-year-old student (Figure 3.4). She will be taking her GCSEs in the summer. Recently she has been suffering from severe headaches which mean that she cannot think clearly enough to complete her coursework. This is putting her under a considerable amount of stress, which she is finding difficult to cope with. She has a very supportive family and group of friends who are doing all they can to help her with these problems.

# Activity

1.  Look at the list of statements about being healthy in Table 3.1 below. For each statement, decide which aspect of health it is most concerned with – physical, intellectual, emotional, or social.

    ▶ Free of pain
    ▶ Coping with stress
    ▶ Having shiny hair and a clear complexion
    ▶ Rarely being ill
    ▶ Living to an old age
    ▶ Being slim
    ▶ Being relaxed and happy
    ▶ Able to play sports
    ▶ Being able to think clearly
    ▶ Having lots of energy
    ▶ Being a non-smoker
    ▶ Rarely going to the doctor
    ▶ Enjoying being with family and friends
    ▶ Helping others

    Adapted from *'Promoting health – a practical guide to health education'*

2.  Read through the case studies on the previous page and following page. Draw Table 3.1 and complete it by adding comments (for example, 'good', 'poor', 'not enough information available to comment') to show how you would assess each of the aspects of their health from the information you have.

| ASPECT OF HEALTH | SHAZIYA | ANDREW | MARIE |
|---|---|---|---|
| ● Physical | | | |
| ● Intellectual | | | |
| ● Emotional | | | |
| ● Social | | | |

Table 3.1 *Complete with comments on the different aspects of health (see case studies)*

CASE STUDY
TWO:
ANDREW

Andrew (Figure 3.5) runs a 150-acre farm single-handedly. Apart from the odd cold, he is rarely ill, and the nature of his work means that he is extremely physically fit. However, over the past few years, the crisis in the beef industry has caused his income to plummet and he is constantly worried because he has fallen behind with his feed bill payments. He does not mind the form-filling that other farmers often complain about, and keeps up to date with his paperwork. He rarely leaves the farm and has no close friends. His elderly father, who was his business partner for a number of years, recently went to live with his sister two hundred miles away.

CASE STUDY
THREE:
MARIE

Marie (Figure 3.6) worked as a nurse in a busy London hospital for a number of years until giving this up when she had her baby, Sam. Her partner works long hours and often travels abroad on business, which means Marie is often alone with Sam. She misses her interesting work and rarely sees her friends. Because Sam often wakes in the night, Marie feels tired all the time. She spends a lot of time just sitting in front of the television, snacking on 'junk' food which has caused her to put on a lot of weight.

People have **different standards** of what being healthy means to them (Figure 3.7). This may depend on:

▶ **Age** – ideas about health and well-being change over time. For example, a young person might only consider themselves healthy if they can take part in active sports, but an elderly person may consider themselves healthy if they can walk a short distance. From middle age onwards, people are more likely to think of mental well-being as well as physical well-being.

## Activity

Read through the following statements, then match each person's definition of health with one of the three types of definition described on page 194 (i.e. negative definition, positive definition or holistic definition).

1. A young mother who is just expecting her third child: 'To me, health is being able to cope with the children.'
2. An elderly man: 'Health is when you haven't got any aches or pains and there's nothing wrong with you.'
3. A twelve year old girl: 'I think that health is about feeling good. You feel strong and happy and relaxed.'

▶ **Sex** – more women than men include social relationships in their definition of health. For example, a woman is more likely to include meeting people, helping people, and having a good relationship with her family when talking about being healthy.

▶ **Lifestyle** – a smoker, for example, may not see a permanent cough as a sign of illness, or an elderly person may think the loss of teeth is normal.

▶ **Class** – studies have shown that middle-class people are more likely to think of health in positive terms, and working-class people are more likely to think of health in negative terms.

▶ **Where a person lives** – people living in an area where many children die within their first year and adults have a short life expectancy will have a different perception of health from people living in an area where death in childhood is rare and adults expect to life to a 'ripe old age'.

▶ **Culture** – people from certain cultures may have ideas about health which are different from a typical Western approach. For example, **Hindus** believe that illness is caused by the elements being out of harmony with the body. Treatment may include diet, massages and herbal cures to restore balance. **Muslims** believe the body has four humours which are out of balance when a person is ill. They may be treated with yoga, diet or massage.

These examples show that ordinary people have a very **subjective** view of health.

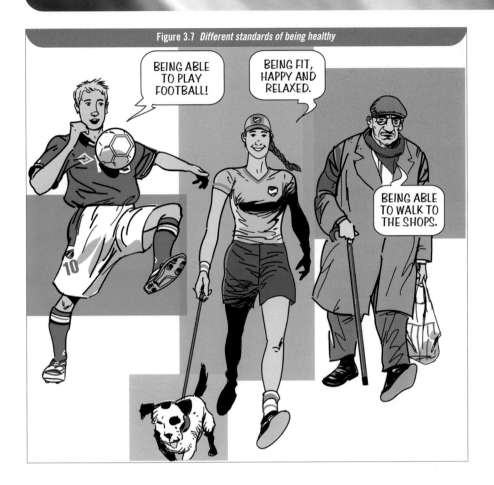

Figure 3.7 *Different standards of being healthy*

# FACTORS POSITIVELY INFLUENCING HEALTH AND WELL-BEING

What factors contribute positively to health and well-being throughout the lifespan?

A person's health and well-being is affected by a number of different factors. Some of the main factors that contribute positively are:

▶ a balanced diet

▶ regular exercise

▶ supportive relationships

▶ adequate financial resources

▶ stimulating work, education and leisure activity

▶ use of health monitoring and illness prevention services (such as screening and vaccination)

▶ use of risk management to protect individuals and promote personal safety.

# Activity

1. A survey on the concept of health asked the following two questions:
   (i) Think of someone you know who is very healthy. Who are you thinking of? How old are they? What makes you call them healthy?
   (ii) At times people are healthier than at other times. What is it like when you are healthy?

   Write down your answers to these questions and then ask a number of other people of different ages these questions and record their answers. Do their answers show that people of different ages have different ideas of what being healthy means?

2. Read the statements listed in Activity 1 on page 200.
   (i) Tick **all** of those that are important to you.
   (ii) Choose the **five** statements which are the **most** important aspects of being healthy to you.
   (iii) Put these five **in order**, starting with the most important aspect.
   (iv) If you are working in a group **compare** your answers with others.
   (v) Now think how an elderly person's answers may differ from yours.

3. Ask a person from each of the following categories to describe how they feel when they are healthy. (Note: you will need to ask a parent or carer to describe a healthy infant.)
   ▶ Infant (0–3 years old)
   ▶ Young children (3–9 years old)
   ▶ Adolescents (10–18 years old)
   ▶ Adults (19–65 years old)
   ▶ Elderly people (65+ years)

   Make a poster to show the different attitudes to health, with a photo of each person and a brief description of their view of being healthy.

## Diet

### A Balanced Diet

*'You are what you eat.'*

*'A good diet is an important way of protecting health.'*

*'Eat yourself fit.'*

These statements indicate the importance of diet to good health. A balanced diet has to contain the following:

- proteins
- carbohydrates
- fats
- fibre
- vitamins
- minerals
- water.

(See Figure 3.8).

### Proteins

Proteins are required for growth and repair. They are major components in the structure of **enzymes** (which control all the chemical reactions within the body), **haemoglobin** (which is the part of the red blood cells that carries oxygen), and cell membranes. Meat, fish, cheese, eggs, nuts, grains and pulses are all good sources of protein.

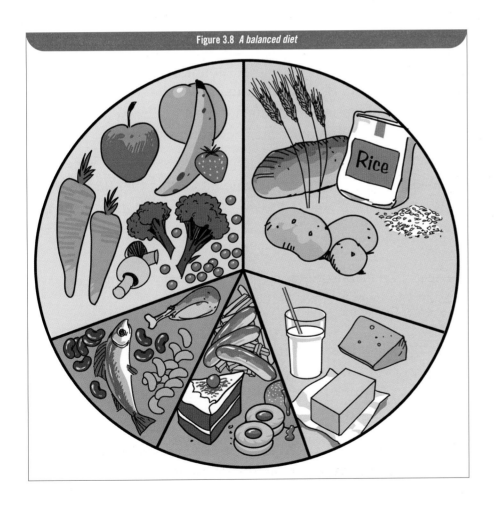

**Figure 3.8 *A balanced diet***

# Activity

1 Find a book or a website which shows the composition of a number of common foods. Which foods are good sources of:

 ▶ protein
 ▶ carbohydrates
 ▶ fats
 ▶ energy?

2 If possible use a computer programme or Internet website to analyse your diet and check that it is balanced. (See the resources listed at the end of the chapter.)

### Carbohydrates

Carbohydrates are the most important source of energy in the diet. Foods that are rich in carbohydrate are those which contain a lot of sugar, such as sweets and cakes, or those which contain a lot of starch, such as pasta, rice and bread. Because **starchy** foods release sugars more slowly and over a longer period of time into the blood, these foods are preferable to **sugary** foods.

### Fats

Fats are a concentrated source of energy. They are necessary to provide us with fat-soluble vitamins, and they are an important component in cell membranes and some hormones. Plants tend to have liquid fats (oils) which are mainly **unsaturated**. Animal fats are solid at room temperature and are mainly **saturated**. (The terms 'saturated' and 'unsaturated' refer to the relative amount of hydrogen in the molecules. It is thought that an excess of saturated fat is particularly harmful to our health.)

### Fibre

There is a type of carbohydrate, known as **cellulose**, which surrounds all plant cells. Cellulose cannot be broken down, so it remains undigested and is eliminated in the faeces. This fibre helps food to keep moving though the gut and prevents constipation. All fruit and vegetables are good sources of fibre.

### Vitamins

Vitamins are essential in small amounts in the diet for maintaining good health. Table 3.2 gives some of their main uses and sources.

### Minerals

We need 15 minerals (or inorganic salts) in our diet. Table 3.3 gives uses and sources of some of these.

### Water

Water is vital for health and is central to a balanced intake. A large proportion of food consists of water, and on top of this a person should aim to drink the equivalent of six to eight cups, mugs, or glasses of fluid a day.

| VITAMIN | SOURCE | METABOLIC FUNCTIONS | EFFECTS OF DEFICIENCY | DAILY REQUIREMENT |
|---|---|---|---|---|
| **Fat-soluble vitamins** | | | | |
| A | liver, green leafy vegetables | provide visual pigment; bone/teeth growth | dry skin, increased susceptibility to resp-iratory/urinary/digestive tract infection, skin sores; 'night blindness'; slow bone/tooth growth | 450 µg |
| D | synthesised in skin using UV light; also in fish liver, fish oils, egg yolk, milk | absorption of calcium and phosphate from gut | demineralisation of bone (rickets in children) | |
| E | Nuts, wheatgerm, seed oils, green leafy vegetables | promotes wound healing and neural function | slow wound healing | |
| K | produced by intestinal bacteria; also in spinach, cauliflower, cabbage, liver | synthesis of blood clotting factors | delayed blood clotting | |
| **Water-soluble vitamins** | | | | |
| $B_1$ (thiamin) | whole grain, eggs, pork, liver, yeast | essential for nerves | energy deficient; partial paralysis of digestive tract/skeletal muscle (beri-beri); degeneration of myelin sheath around nerve cells | 400 µg |
| B2 (riboflavin) | yeast, liver, beef, lamb, eggs, whole grain, peas, peanuts; small quantities produced by gut bacteria | for release of energy from food | deficiency signs rarely seen | 1.0 µg |
| $B_3$ (niacin or nicotinamide) | yeast, meats, liver, fish, whole grain, peas, beans | for release of energy from food. | pellagra (skin disease) diarrhoea | 5.5 µg |
| $B_{12}$ | liver, kidney, milk, eggs, cheese, meats | cell division | anaemia; | 1.25 µg |
| Folate (folic acid) | green leafy vegetables, liver; synthesised by gut bacteria | red/white blood cell production | amaemia due to abnormally large red blood cells; neural tube abnormality in foetus | 150 µg |
| C (ascorbic acid) | citrus fruits, tomatoes, green vegetables | formation of connective tissue and wound healing | retarded growth; poor connective tissue repair/growth (scurvy) including swollen gums, toothe loosening, fragile blood vessels; poor wound healing | 25 µg **NB** 1000 µg = 1 mg |

Table 3.2 *The sources and uses of vitamins*

| MINERAL | SOURCE | FUNCTION | DAILY REQUIREMENT | EFFECTS OF DEFICIENCY |
|---------|--------|----------|-------------------|------------------------|
| calcium | milk, egg yolk, shellfish, green leafy vegetables | formation of bones/teeth; blood clotting, muscle contraction; cell division | 700 mg | loss of bone density, e.g. osteomalacia/ rickets |
| potassium | widespread | action potential of muscle/nerve cells | 3500 mg | |
| sodium | widespread – table salt | water balance of body muscle nerve function | 1600 mg | |
| magnesium | beans, peanuts, bananas | role in bone formation and muscle/nerve cell functions: release of energy from food | 1.4 mg | muscle weakness; convulsions; hypertension |
| iron | widespread but esp. red meats, liver, beans, fruits, nuts, legumes | component of haemoglobin; component of chemicals involved in cell respiration | 8.7 mg | anaemia |
| iodine (iodide) | seafood, cod-liver oil, iodised table salt | component of thyroid hormones | 140 µg | thyroid hormone deficiency (induces thyroid goitre) |
| zinc | widespread but esp. meats | component of some enzymes; promotes normal growth, involved in taste and appetite; sperm production | 8.5 mg | dermatitis; growth retardation; diarrhoea |
| copper | eggs, wholewheat flour, liver, fish, spinach | haemoglobin synthesis; component of some enzymes | 1.2 mg | retarded growth; cerebral degeneration |
| chromium | yeast, beer, beef | involved in insulin synthesis | 25 µg | |

Table 3.3 Sources and uses of minerals

## Recommended daily amounts of the different food groups

The amount of energy (in carbohydrates and fat), protein, vitamins and minerals required each day depends on factors such as our level of activity and age.

### *How much protein do we need?*

The average UK diet provides more than enough protein: men generally consume 85 grams of protein a day, and women consume 62 grams. The recommended intake for an adult is 0.75 grams of protein per kilogram of body weight per day. (For example, a person weighing 70 kg would require 0.75 X 70 grams of protein per day.) Some people, however, require additional supplies of protein, such as growing children and babies; pregnant or lactating mothers; people who exercise heavily; people with viral infections such as measles, because protein is lost from their muscles, and is also needed for their immune defence; and patients who are recovering from illness or surgery.

### *How much vitamins and minerals do we need?*

Tables 3.2 and 3.3 show the daily requirements of vitamins and minerals.

## Activity

Figure 3.9 shows the energy needs of different individuals. Look at the graph and list three factors that affect our energy requirements. (Answers on page 273).

## Activity

Use Figure 3.10 to calculate how many grams of protein you should consume each day. (You will need to multiply the recommended amount for your age group by your body weight.)

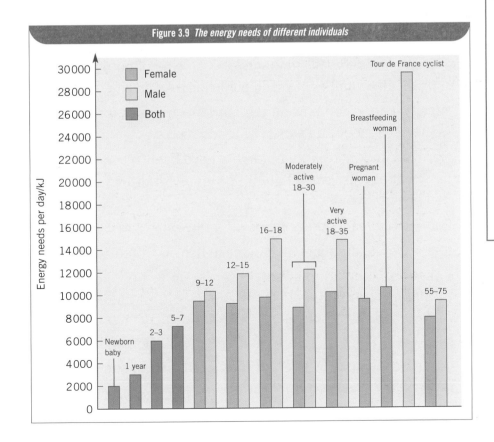

**Figure 3.9** *The energy needs of different individuals*

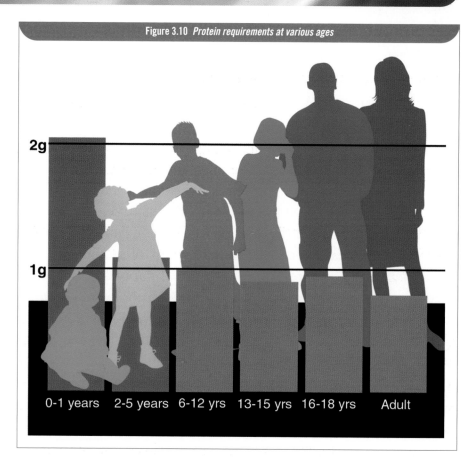

**Figure 3.10** *Protein requirements at various ages*

2g

1g

0-1 years    2-5 years    6-12 yrs    13-15 yrs    16-18 yrs    Adult

## Healthy eating – ten top tips

Because it is difficult for people to estimate whether they are having their recommended daily amounts of each type of nutrient in their diet, there are a number of useful guidelines worth remembering.

▶ No single food contains all the nutrients we need for health, so we need to eat a wide variety of foods each day.

▶ National and international targets have been set to encourage us to eat at least five 80 gram portions of fruit and vegetables every day.

▶ Eat lots of bread, other cereals or potatoes.

▶ Eat moderate amounts of lean meat, fish and alternatives.

▶ Eat moderate amounts of lower-fat milk and dairy foods (although children under two years old should not have reduced-fat milk.)

▶ An average adult should drink about six to eight cups of liquid a day. (For example, water, fruit juice, skimmed or semi-skimmed milk, or low sugar soft drinks.)

▶ Avoid eating too much fat and fatty food, particularly saturated fats.

▶ Eat sparingly foods containing sugar.

▶ Use a minimum amount of salt in cooking and try not to add additional salt.

▶ Healthy food needn't be boring. A balanced diet can contain chips and chocolate – it's just a matter of getting the balance right.

## Special Diets

The information above on recommended daily amounts of each type of nutrient shows that certain groups of people have particular dietary requirements.

### Babies

If possible, the best way to provide a baby with food is by **breast feeding**. Breast milk contains all the nutrients necessary for the first few months of a baby's life in the most easily digestible form. It will also protect the baby against some diseases as it contains antibodies, and may help establish a close bond between the mother and baby. Breastfeeding is more economical and convenient than bottle feeding, as the milk is always at the correct temperature and there is no equipment to sterilise (Figure 3.11.)

However, it is sometimes not possible for a baby to be breastfed, and the baby will be **bottle-fed** with **specially formulated baby milk**. It is important that this milk is made up according to the instructions on the tin or packet. It is recommended that cows' milk is not given to babies until they are at least one year old. **Solid food** can be introduced when the baby is between four and six months old, with breastfeeding or bottle feeding continuing.

### Children

It is particularly important that children have a well-balanced diet because childhood is a period of active growth and development. There is also evidence that if a child develops healthy eating habits, these will last into adulthood. Children have a high protein requirement for growth (Figure 3.10) and a high energy requirement relative to their small size. Their diet should be low in salt because their kidneys are unable to cope with high amounts. It can be difficult to feed 'fussy' children, but the following make healthy snacks:

▶ fresh or dried fruit

▶ raw vegetables, like carrots

## Activity

Produce a leaflet or poster aimed at a new parent on one of the following topics:
▶ breastfeeding
▶ bottle-feeding with formulated baby milk
▶ introducing solid food into a baby's diet.

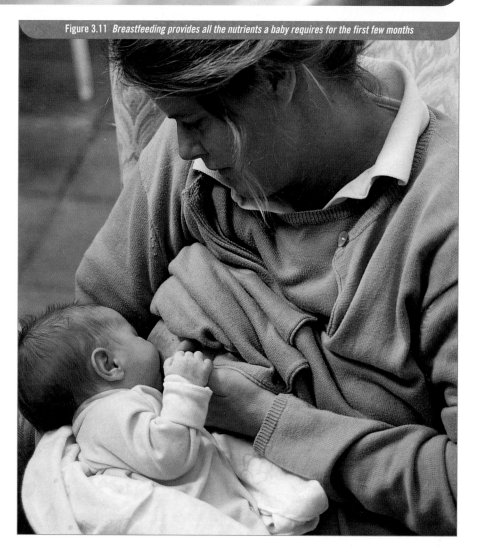

Figure 3.11 *Breastfeeding provides all the nutrients a baby requires for the first few months*

- bread or unsweetened biscuits
- unsweetened breakfast cereals (with milk, or dry)
- popcorn.

### Pregnant and breastfeeding women

In the womb the developing baby obtains all its nutrients from the mother. It is, therefore, very important that she has a balanced diet. However, if the mother's diet is lacking in some way, this is more likely to harm the mother's health than the baby's health. For example, if the mother's diet lacks iron, the mother will become anaemic but the baby will not. If the mother's diet lacks calcium, the baby's bones will develop normally, but this will use up much of the calcium in the mother's bones, causing them to become softer, or even bent.

A woman should gain only 9–13 kg during the whole of her pregnancy. This means that while pregnant there is no need for her to eat more than usual. What is important is that she takes care to eat a balanced diet. It is necessary for pregnant women to have adequate fibre in their diet, because the hormones produced in pregnancy may lead to constipation.

Women need a higher level of extra nutrients when they are breastfeeding than when they are pregnant. For example, they require more protein, vitamins and iron. The fat which accumulates in the woman's body during pregnancy can be broken down to produce some of the extra energy needed for milk production, but they will also need a more energy-rich diet.

## Activity

1   There is currently a debate about whether the government should make it compulsory for folic acid to be added to all manufactured bread and cakes. High levels are required in the first month after conception to prevent babies being born with neural tube defects, such as spina bifida. It may also cut heart disease, and there are no apparent harmful side effects. If you have the opportunity, divide into two groups (one **for** compulsory addition of folic acid, and one **against**), spend some time preparing your arguments, and then debate the issue.

2   If possible, speak to a mother who has breastfed her baby. Find out if her normal diet changed when she was breastfeeding. For example, did she have a higher calorific intake?

### The elderly

As people get older their energy requirement drops, partly because their metabolic rate decreases, and partly because they are likely to exercise less. However, it is important that the diet is not neglected in old age and that, even if the quantity eaten decreases, the quality and nutrient content of food remains high. Vitamin C deficiency is quite common in this age group due to a lack of fresh fruit and vegetables in the diet.

## Activity

List the reasons you can think of for why older people may neglect their diet. (Answers on page 273.) Suggest ways in which the elderly could be encouraged to eat a healthy diet.

# Regular exercise

Regular exercise can have a very positive effect on health at any age. Some of the physical effects of exercise are listed below, but it should be remembered that any recreation undertaken in a group can also be good for a person's social health, and that exercising can lift feelings of mild depression, improve self-esteem, improve alertness and reduce stress. The degree to which physical activity affects the body depends on:

▶ the type of exercise and how vigorous it is
▶ the duration of the exercise
▶ the number of times a week the exercise is repeated
▶ how fit the person is already.

The latest research shows that 30 minutes of brisk physical activity five times a week are needed to improve health. This means any activity which makes you slightly out of breath. People who are not used to exercise should start with less and gradually build up to this.

## Physical effects of exercise

▶ The heart becomes more efficient.
▶ Blood volume, red cells and haemoglobin increase.
▶ Arteries grow larger.
▶ Diaphragm grows stronger.
▶ Lungs become more expandable and increase in volume.
▶ Co-ordination improves.
▶ The muscles and tendons can be stretched more easily, thus increasing flexibility of joints.
▶ Muscles increase in strength.
▶ It prevents obesity.
▶ The immune system produces more white blood cells to help fight infection.
▶ The chances of developing conditions like arthritis, high blood pressure, diabetes, stroke, osteoporosis (brittle bone disease) or heart disease later in life are reduced.
▶ The effects of ageing are reduced.

## Children and exercise

The amount of exercise children take has declined over recent decades. This has been caused partly by the increase in the amount of television watched, and partly because parents allow children to play outside less because of the increase in the amount of traffic. It should be remembered that taking part in games and sports helps children to develop friendships and self-esteem, and so has a positive effect on their social, emotional and intellectual health, as well as on their physical health. It is important that children have positive role models. For example, it has been found that more active parents tend to have more active children.

## Teenagers and exercise

During adolescence, physical activity declines by almost 50%, with females reducing their exercise levels even more than males. By the time they are 18, fewer than 12% of people take enough exercise to be considered fit.

## Pregnant women and exercise

Studies have shown that exercising during pregnancy is beneficial to the woman's health, and does no harm to the baby. It can reduce the mother's discomfort, tone the muscles in preparation for childbirth, improve her emotional health, and help with the control of weight gain. However, the following precautions should be taken by pregnant women.

▶ Check with your doctor before starting an exercise programme.

▶ Exercise at moderate intensity for 20 to 30 minutes at least three times a week.

▶ Don't exercise on your back after the first three months. This could reduce blood flow to your and your baby's heart.

▶ Avoid sudden-stop sports like tennis, or sports in which you may fall.

▶ Call your doctor if you feel faint, sick, short of breath, or have abdominal pain or vaginal bleeding.

## Elderly people and exercise

Exercise is effective in slowing down the physical decline associated with ageing. For example, elderly people who exercise have significantly lower blood pressure and better balance than those who do not exercise. They also sleep better. Swimming is considered a particularly good exercise because it works every muscle in the body without stressing joints. Some elderly people take part in very active sports, but it should be remembered that effective exercise can even be taken when sitting in a chair. Exercise done as a member of a group can have a positive effect on physical, social, emotional and intellectual health (Figure 3.12.)

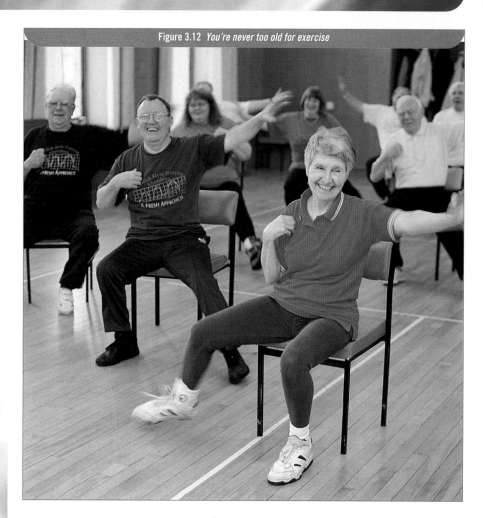
Figure 3.12 *You're never too old for exercise*

## Activity

1   Look at the recommended amount of exercise above (5 × 30 min. each week). If you are not already doing this amount, plan activities that you would enjoy doing and see how you could fit these into your week. (**NB** Even short bursts of activity for 10 minutes or so add up to make a significant difference to your fitness.)

2   Find out if there are any exercise classes in your area aimed specifically at the elderly. If you go out on work experience to a local day or residential centre for the elderly, find out what opportunities for exercise are offered.

### Individuals with special needs

People with disabilities can take part in a wide variety of sports (Figure 3.13).

### Danger: too much exercise!

Many athletes train at a level which is harmful to their health. If too much exercise is undertaken, there is a higher risk of sports-related injuries, and research has shown that there may be a higher rate of infection. Very intensive exercise can delay puberty. Some people are thought to become addicted to exercise, which means that lack of physical activity will have an adverse effect on their mental health.

## Supportive relationships

Read the following sections:

▶   The effects of relationships on personal development (Chapter 3, page 300)

▶   Social isolation (page 246).

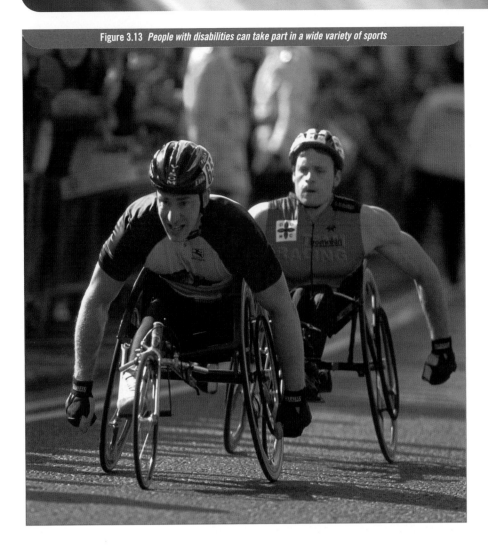

Figure 3.13 *People with disabilities can take part in a wide variety of sports*

# Activity

The following relationships may contribute positively to health and well-being:

▶ family relationships (for example, with parents, siblings, children)
▶ friendships
▶ intimate personal and sexual relationships
▶ working relationships (including teacher/student, employer/employee, peers, colleagues).

Think of examples of relationships you have with specific people and describe how they contribute positively to your health and well-being.

# Adequate financial support

An adequate income is needed to ensure that a number of requirements for good health are met. It will allow a person to have:

▶ a healthy diet (see page 202)

▶ satisfactory housing (see page 249)

▶ stimulating education and leisure activities (below)

▶ lower stress levels.

The section on *Poverty* (pages 248) explains how the lack of adequate financial resources can adversely affect health and well-being.

# Stimulating work, education and leisure activity

Work, education and leisure activities can contribute positively to all aspects of health and well-being – physical, intellectual, emotional and social. These activities can all provide supportive relationships, and help to prevent social isolation (see page 246). Work can provide adequate financial resources, and prevent poverty (see page 248). The risks to health from unemployment are described on page 251.

Education has been said to be 'the one way out of the dismal mixture of poverty, unemployment and crime' (Figure 3.14). People with very low literacy are much more likely to be classified as depressed than those with good basic skills. Good education can improve health on two fronts. It can inform pupils and students

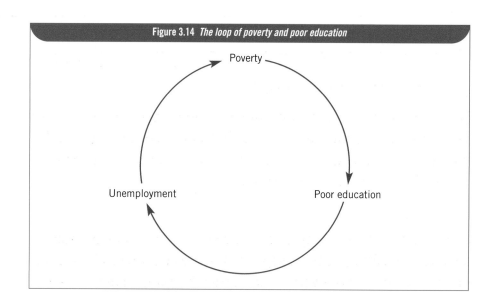

**Figure 3.14** *The loop of poverty and poor education*

about health-related topics, such as diet and teenage pregnancy, and it can improve a person's chances of employment and, therefore, make them less likely to suffer from poverty.

# Activity

1.  (i)  In 1997 the Government Minister for Public Health said schools could do more to help health and well-being. It was suggested that schools should develop a 'healthy school' philosophy and, for example, put more emphasis on supplying healthy school meals, and reducing teenage pregnancies.

    In what ways do you think your school helps its students' health and well-being?

    In what ways do you think your school could do more to help its students' health and well-being?

    (ii) *The Minister for Health also said 'Teenage pregnancy is all too likely to be a cause as well as a symptom of poor education, unemployment and social exclusion. If a healthy school can keep a child from following her mother by getting pregnant at 17, she has a better chance of getting qualifications, getting a job, and breaking out of the loop.'*

    How do you think teenage pregnancy can **cause** poor education? (Answers on page 273).

    Do you agree that teenage pregnancy is likely to be a **symptom** of poor education (i.e. that a girl with a poor education is more likely to get pregnant as a teenager than a girl who has received a better education)?

2.  If you have experience of **employment**, write down what you gained from this, other than pay. If you have not been employed, informally interview people who are, and ask them how they feel they benefit from employment, other than financially. (Answers on page 273).

# Use of health monitoring and illness prevention services

The increase in health monitoring and illness prevention services has led to an improvement in health. Health monitoring includes the use of **screening**, and illness prevention services include **vaccination**. These are described below.

## Screening

A screening test is a simple test carried out on a large number of apparently healthy people to separate those who probably have a certain disease from those who do not. Screening programmes can be:

- for **specific groups**, for example for pregnant women, newborn babies, children, women, men, or older people
- for **particular diseases**, for example, breast cancer.

### *Advantages of screening*

- Individuals can make more informed choices about their health.
- Treatment can be given before a person shows signs of ill health.
- Screening can reduce the risk of a person developing a condition or its complications.
- Screening has the potential to save lives or improve the quality of life.

### *Disadvantages of screening*

- Screening cannot guarantee protection against a disease.
- People will occasionally be told they have the condition when they don't (**false positive results**).
- People will occasionally be told they don't have the condition when they do (**false negative results**).

### *Examples of screening programmes*

#### Antenatal screening

In the UK all women are offered a test for:

- rubella antibodies (to check if they are immune to German measles)
- syphilis
- HIV
- hepatitis B.

Screening is only performed with the mother's consent.

#### Neonatal screening

All babies are examined as soon as possible after the birth. Screening tests are carried out to check for specific disorders that can be successfully treated if detected early enough. They include tests for:

- congenital dislocation of the hip
- phenylketonuria (PKU)
- thyroid function.

There are plans to introduce a test for cystic fibrosis in the future.

## Childhood screening

Over the first few years of a child's life a number of other conditions will be checked for, for example, tests will be made for:

▶ cataracts

▶ congenital heart defects

▶ normal hearing.

### Breast cancer screening for women

Women are first invited for this type of screening between their 50th and 53rd birthday. In 2000–2001, 75% of those invited were screened. Altogether 1.3 million women of all ages were screened and 8345 cases of cancer were diagnosed.

### Cervical cancer screening

Women are invited for this type of screening every three to four years from the age of 20. In 2000–2001, 3.6 million women were screened in the UK. The test involves the collection of a sample of cells from the cervix (neck of the womb). These are then examined under a microscope for abnormalities.

## Vaccination

When bacteria or viruses enter the body, the immune system makes **antibodies** to destroy them. These antibodies are proteins that stick to the invader and destroy it. The immune response can be artificially induced by vaccination. When the vaccine is given it stimulates the production of antibodies without actually causing the disease. This means that later, when an individual comes into contact with the disease, there will be a rapid response and the bacteria and viruses will quickly be killed.

There are a number of different types of vaccine.

▶ **Live attenuated vaccine** – this is a very weak preparation of a living, disease-causing organism.

▶ **Inactivated vaccine** – this is a preparation of dead disease-causing organisms.

▶ **Extracts of toxins** – this is a preparation of poisonous substances from the bacteria, which has been made harmless.

The above methods produce what is known as **active immunity**. This means they cause the individual to produce their own antibodies. **Passive immunity** involves acquiring antibodies, not making them. Antibodies from other people or mammals, for example, horses, can be injected. Passive immunity gives more

> ## Activity
>
> The UK National Screening Committee advises the Government on all aspects of screening policy. Have a look at their website which explains how screening programmes work.

immediate protection than active immunity, because there is no delay while the person's immune system makes antibodies. However, passive immunity only lasts as long as the antibodies, which is usually just a few weeks.

Vaccination is available against:

- diphtheria
- whooping cough
- tetanus
- poliomyelitis
- measles
- tuberculosis (TB)
- mumps
- rubella
- influenza
- hepatitis A and B
- rabies
- cholera
- typhoid
- anthrax
- smallpox
- yellow fever.

### *Vaccination programmes in the UK*

- **Children** are routinely vaccinated against diphtheria, whooping cough, tetanus, poliomyelitis and measles.

- The BCG vaccination is used to prevent tuberculosis, but often people pick up a mild form of this and develop their own immunity naturally.

- All **girls** should be vaccinated against rubella (German measles) between their tenth and fourteenth birthday.

Figure 3.15 shows the increase in immunisation rates over the past two decades. As the immunisation rate has increased, there has been a corresponding fall in the relevant diseases, for example, German measles has been almost eradicated from Britain and America. There were no recorded cases in Britain in the last quarter of 2000. Figure 3.16 shows the decrease in measles cases after the introduction of the measles vaccination.

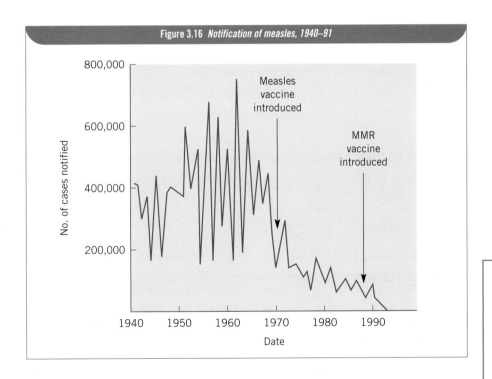

Figure 3.15  *The immunisation uptake rate, England 1983–2000*

Community Health and Prevention: Vaccination and immunisation
England                                                                 **Numbers and percentages**

| | 1993–94 | 1994–95 | 1995–96 | 1996–97 | 1997–98 | 1998–99 | 1999–2000 |
|---|---|---|---|---|---|---|---|
| **Percentage of children immunised by their 2nd birthday** | | | | | | | |
| Diphtheria/tetanus/polio | 95 | 95 | 96 | 96 | 96 | 95 | 95 |
| Pertussis (whooping cough) | 93 | 93 | 94 | 94 | 94 | 94 | 94 |
| Measles/mumps/rubella | 91 | 91 | 92 | 92 | 91 | 88 | 88 |
| Haemophilus influenzae b | 75 | 91 | 94 | 95 | 95 | 95 | 94 |
| **BCG vaccinations by age (thousands)** | | | | | | | |
| under 1 | 47 | 53 | 56 | 64 | 65 | 68 | 61 |
| 1–9 | 6 | 5 | 6 | 6 | 6 | 5 | 4 |
| 10–15 | 409 | 256 | 509 | 407 | 442 | 395 | 129 |
| 16 & over | 6 | 4 | 5 | 6 | 5 | 7 | 3 |

• The proportion of children who have been immunised by their second birthday against diptheria, tetanus and polio rose in 1995–96 to 96%, the highest ever recorded.
• Uptake of immunisation against pertussis and of immunisation against haemophilus influenzae b reached 95% in 1996–97.

Figure 3.16  *Notification of measles, 1940–91*

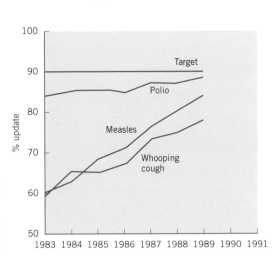

Recent controversy over the perceived risk of giving children the MMR vaccination is discussed in the section on risk management, below.

## Activity

1. Have you been tested for natural immunity to tuberculosis? If so, describe how was this done.
2. Why are girls vaccinated against German measles, but not boys?

(Answer on page 273.)

# Use of risk management to protect individuals and promote personal safety

▶ A **hazard** is defined as anything that has the potential to cause harm.

▶ A **risk** is how likely it is that a hazard will cause actual harm.

▶ **Risk management** is action taken to minimise risks.

Health and safety at work legislation is in place to protect individuals and promote personal safety in the workplace. However, as the article below shows, people are at greater risk from accidents in the home.

Health decisions sometimes need to be taken by professionals and by individuals in which risks have to be compared. Recently there has been controversy over the use of the MMR vaccine (see above). Although there is no scientific evidence to support it, some parents are concerned that the MMR (triple) vaccine can cause some children to develop autism. Some parents have chosen for their children to have separate vaccines for each disease. However, this means total immunity may be delayed, and some children may not receive all the necessary injections. Some parents have chosen not to have their children vaccinated at all. Once the level of vaccination in a population drops below a certain level, there is a high risk of an epidemic occurring (see the article from the Daily Telegraph below). Parents therefore have to balance the perceived risk of autism with the risk of measles.

**Figure 3.17** *An article from the Guardian, 20/3/01*

## Home accidents kill 76 a week

More people are killed in the home every week – an average of 76 – than die in road accidents (66), government figures reveal today. The causes included fires, carbon monoxide poisoning, burns, drowning, and DIY accidents. In 1999 more than 2.8m people needed hospital treatment following domestic accidents.

**Figure 3.18** *An article from the Daily Telegraph, 2/2/02*

## MMR-free nursery hit by measles outbreak
### By Andrew Hibberd

Three children from a private nursery have contracted measles and 22 others have been tested for the disease.

None of the infected children had received the controversial MMR (measles, mumps and rubella) triple vaccine despite recent attempts by the Department of Health to assure parents that it is safe.

The measles outbreak has been confirmed at a time when Public Health Laboratory Service figures show national take-up of the MMR vaccine between July and September last year fell to a record low of 84.2 per cent, a long way short of the 95 per cent target. A spokesperson said: "This is the lowest we have seen for the UK since monitoring started in 1995."

**Figure 3.19** *An article from The Times, 6/2/02*

## SUNBEDS DOUBLE THE RISK OF SKIN CANCER

**By Mark Henderson**

*Science Correspondent*

Sunbeds and tanning lamps may be causing thousands of cases of skin cancer every year, scientists say.

Research in the United States has shown that people who have used artificial tanning devices are up to 2.5 times more likely to develop certain kinds of skin cancer than those who have never visited a tanning salon. The risks are greatest in the young, with the chances of developing a tumour increasing by up to 20 per cent for each decade of sunbed use before the age of 50. Young women are by far the most likely people to seek an artificial tan.

## Activity

Read the article on the left. If you regularly used a sunbed, would this article influence your behaviour?

# RISKS TO HEALTH AND WELL-BEING

There are a number of factors that put an individual's health and well-being at risk. Some of these are lifestyle factors over which a person has control; others are genetic, social and economic factors over which a person has no control. The risks to health and well-being explained below are:

▶ genetically inherited diseases and conditions

▶ substance misuse (including misuse of legal and illegal drugs, solvents, tobacco smoking, and excessive alcohol intake)

▶ an unbalanced, poor quality or inadequate diet

▶ too much stress

▶ lack of personal hygiene

▶ lack of regular physical exercise

▶ unprotected sex

▶ social isolation

▶ poverty

▶ inadequate housing

▶ unemployment

▶ environmental pollution.

## Genetically inherited diseases and conditions

Certain diseases are carried in a person's genetic material (DNA) and can be passed from parent to child.

- There are over 4000 recognised genetic diseases
- A baby is born in the UK with a genetic disease or birth defect, on average, every 26 minutes.

Examples of genetically inherited diseases and conditions include:

- sickle cell anaemia
- haemophilia
- Huntington's chorea
- cystic fibrosis
- Down's syndrome.

The effect of these diseases on health and well-being varies from condition to condition, and person to person. A person suffering from a genetic disorder may suffer mild symptoms intermittently, or may be severely disabled with a short life expectancy.

There are a number of screening methods that can be used to detect a genetic disorder in an unborn baby.

- A pregnant woman will be offered a specialised **blood test**, which can indicate the risk of her baby having Down's syndrome.

- An **ultrasound test**, in which the tissues of the body are imaged using sound waves, can also indicate if there is a risk that the baby may have Down's syndrome.

- If blood tests (see above) indicate that a woman has an increased risk of having a baby with Down's syndrome, or if there is a family history of a genetic disorder, **amniocentesis** will be offered. This involves inserting a fine needle through the abdominal wall into the uterus and taking a sample of the amniotic fluid that surrounds the foetus. This sample contains cells from the baby. The cells can be grown and the chromosomes can be examined for genetic disorders.

- Cells from the foetus can also be taken from the placenta, a technique known as **chorionic villus sampling**.

If a genetic disorder is detected, the mother will be offered a termination.

There are few examples of a genetic disease being cured. The cases that have been successful have involved children who suffer from a genetic disorder that affects their immune system. This means that they are often ill with infections and may not live to adulthood. It is possible to give these children a bone marrow transplant. If successful, they are cured and can then produce the cells needed to fight infection. It is hoped that, in the future, **gene therapy**, where people who lack the healthy gene can be given a replacement gene, will offer hope to individuals suffering from genetic disorders.

# Substance misuse

## Use of illegal drugs

Illegal drugs are those whose non-medicinal use is banned by the *Misuse of Drugs Act*. Table 3.4 gives information on the most commonly used of these. *The Misuse of Drugs Act* places banned drugs in different classes, A, B and C. Offences involving Class A drugs carry the highest penalties; offences involving Class C drugs the lowest.

Almost one in six young people take illegal drugs on a regular basis, according to a recent survey, and almost half of all young people have taken drugs at some time in their life. The survey showed that men aged between 16 and 29 who drink and smoke heavily, are unemployed, and go out a lot in the evenings are most likely to take illegal drugs.

It can be very difficult to tell if a person is using drugs. Signs that parents are encouraged to look out for include the following:

▶ sudden changes of mood from happy and alert to sullen and moody

▶ unusual irritability or aggression

▶ loss of appetite

▶ loss of interest in hobbies, sport, schoolwork or friends

▶ bouts of drowsiness or sleepiness

▶ increased evidence of telling lies or furtive behaviour

▶ unexplained loss of money or belongings from the home

▶ unusual smells, stains, or marks on the body or clothes, or around the house.

(**NB**. Some of these signs are a normal part of growing up, and it is important that people do not jump to conclusions.)

It is difficult to describe the exact effects of a drug because the effect is influenced by:

▶ the amount taken

▶ how much the user has taken before

▶ what the user wants and expects to happen

▶ the surroundings in which it is taken

▶ the reactions of other people.

## Activity

Choose an inherited disease or condition and find out about its:

▶ genetic cause

▶ symptoms

▶ treatment

▶ prognosis.

If working in a group, each person can choose a different disease and then present their findings.

A person who feels they need to keep taking a drug is known as **drug dependent**. This dependence may be either **physical** or **psychological**.

▶ **Physical dependence** – withdrawal from the drug involves physical discomfort.

▶ **Psychological dependence** – withdrawal from the drug results in craving or emotional distress. This is the most widespread and important type of dependence.

Illegal drug use can be particularly harmful to a developing foetus. The unborn baby can be harmed in the following ways.

▶ Drug use affecting the mother's health, either directly or through self-neglect and poor nutrition.

▶ Drugs may directly affect the foetus through the mother's blood stream.

There are particular risks associated with the injection of drugs:

▶ infection may result from the use of non-sterile needles (for example, the transmission of HIV or hepatitis)

▶ abscesses and gangrene may be caused by missing the vein when injecting

▶ dependence is more likely.

Figure 3.20 shows some of the reasons for drug taking.

There is a wide variety of help available for people with drug problems. Details of the services available can be obtained from the National Drugs Helpline (see the *Resources* section at the end of the chapter.) These services are provided by the NHS and voluntary organisations and can link in with other services, such as social care, housing or legal advice. The type of help available includes:

▶ information about drugs

▶ support for drug users and their families

▶ out-patient clinics for treating drug users (e.g. the prescription of illegal drug substitutes)

▶ in-patient treatment for more serious complications

▶ residential rehabilitation services to help people recover from their dependency.

## Activity

1 What advice would you give to a parent who finds out that their child is using illegal drugs?

2 Find out what to do if you were to find someone very drowsy or unconscious because of drug taking. (Answers given on page 273)

3 Look at Table 3.4, which lists a number of illegal drugs. Discuss which age groups are most likely to use each drug.

| | Other names include | What it looks like & how it is taken | The effects |
|---|---|---|---|
| Alkyl nitrites | poppers<br>amyl nitrite, butyl nitrite, isobutyl nitrite<br>product names include:<br>Ram, Thrust, Rock Hard, Kix, TNT, Liquid Gold | • clear or straw-coloured liquid in a small bottle<br>• vapour which is breathed in through the mouth or nose from a small bottle or tube | • brief but intense 'head-rush'<br>• flushed face and neck<br>• effects fade after 2 to 5 minutes |
| Amphetamines | speed, whizz, uppers, amph, billy, sulphate | • grey or white powder that is snorted, swallowed, smoked, injected or dissolved in a drink<br>• tablets which are swallowed | • excitement – the mind races and users feel confident and energetic |
| Cannabis | marijuana, draw, blow, weed, puff, shit, hash, ganja, spliff, wacky backy<br>*Cannabis is the most commonly used drug among 11 to 25 year olds* | • a solid, dark lump known as 'resin'<br>• leaves, stalks and seeds called 'grass'<br>• a sticky, dark oil<br>• can be rolled (usually with tobacco) in a spliff or joint, smoked on its own in a special pipe, or cooked and eaten in food | • users feel relaxed and talkative<br>• cooking the drug then eating it makes the effects more intense and harder to control<br>• may bring on a craving for food (this is often referred to as having the 'munchies') |
| Ecstasy | E, doves, XTC, disco biscuits, echoes, hug drug, burgers, fantasy<br>chemical name: MDMA (currently many tablets contain MDEA, MDA, MBDB)<br>*4% of 16 to 25s have used ecatasy in the last 3 months* | tablets of different shapes, size and colour (but often white) which are swallowed | • users feel alert and in tune with their surroundings<br>• sound, colour and emotions seem much more intense<br>• users may dance for hours<br>• the effects last from 3 to 6 hours |
| Gases, Glues & Aerosols | products such as lighter gas refills, aerosols containing products such as hairspray, deodorants and air fresheners, tins or tubes of glue, some paints, thinners and correcting fluids | • sniffed or breathed into the lungs from a cloth or sleeve<br>• gas products are sometimes squirted directly into the back of the throat | • effects feel similar to being very drunk<br>• users feel thick-headed, dizzy, giggly and dreamy<br>• users may hallucinate<br>• effects don't last very long, but users can remain intoxicated all day by repeating the dose |
| Heroin | smack, brown, horse, gear, junk, H, jack, scag | brownish-white powder which is smoked, snorted or dissolved and injected | • small doses give the user a sense of warmth and well-being<br>• larger doses can make them drowsy and relaxed |
| LSD | acid, trips, tabs, blotters, microdots, dots | 1/4 inch squares of paper, often with a picture on one side, which are swallowed. Microdots and dots are tiny tablets | • effects are known as a 'trip' and can last for 8 to 12 hours<br>• users will experience their surroundings in a very different way<br>• sense of movement and time may speed up or slow down<br>• objects colours and sounds may be distorted |

Table 3.4 *Facts about drugs*

| The health risks | Legal status |
|---|---|
| <ul><li>headache, feeling faint and sick</li><li>regular use can cause skin problems around the mouth and nose</li><li>dangerous for people with anaemia, glaucoma, and breathing or heart problems</li><li>if spilled, can burn the skin</li><li>may be fatal if swallowed</li><li>mixing Viagra with alkyl nitrites may increase the risk of heart problems</li></ul> | <ul><li>amyl nitrite is a prescription-only medicine</li><li>possession is not illegal, but supply can be an offence</li></ul> |
| <ul><li>while on the drug, some users become tense and anxious</li><li>leaves users feeling tired and depressed for one or two days and sometimes longer</li><li>high doses repeated over a few days may cause panic and hallucinations</li><li>long-term use puts a strain on the heart</li><li>heavy, long-term use can lead to mental illness</li><li>mixing Viagra with amphetamines may increase the risk of heart problems</li></ul> | class B (but class A if prepared for injection) |
| <ul><li>smoking it with tobacco may lead to users becoming hooked on cigarettes</li><li>impairs the ability to learn and concentrate</li><li>can leave people tired and lacking energy</li><li>users may lack motivation and feel apathetic</li><li>can make users paranoid and anxious, depending on their mood and situation</li><li>smoking joints over a long period of time can lead to respiratory disorders, including lung cancer</li></ul> | class B (but class A penalties can apply to cannabis oil) |
| <ul><li>can leave users feeling tired and depressed for days</li><li>risk of overheating and dehydration if users dance energetically without taking breaks or drinking enough fluids (users should sip about a pint of non-alcholic fluid such as fruit juice, sports drinks or water every hour)</li><li>use has been linked to liver and kidney problems</li><li>some experts are concerned that use of ecstasy can lead to brain damage causing depression in later life</li><li>mixing Viagra with ecstasy may increase the risk of heart problems</li></ul> | Class A<br>other drugs similar to ecstasy are also illegal and class A |
| <ul><li>nausea, vomiting, black-outs and heart problems that can be fatal</li><li>squirting gas products down the throat may cause the body to produce fluid that floods the lungs and this can cause instant death</li><li>risk of suffocation if the substance is inhaled from a plastic bag over the head</li><li>accidents can happen when the user is high because their senses are affected</li><li>long-term abuse of glue can damage the brain, liver and kidneys</li></ul> | it is illegal for shopkeepers to sell to under-18s, or to people acting for them, it they suspect the product is intended for abuse |
| <ul><li>heroin is addictive (even when smoked)</li><li>users who form a habit may end up taking the drug just to feel normal</li><li>excessive amounts can result in overdose, coma and in some cases death</li><li>injecting can damage veins</li><li>sharing injecting equipment puts users at risk of dangerous infections like hepatitis B or C and HIV/AIDS</li></ul> | Class A |
| <ul><li>once a trip starts it cannot be stopped</li><li>users may have a 'bad trip', which can be terrifying</li><li>'flashbacks' may be experienced where parts of a trip are re-lived some time after the event</li><li>can complicate mental health problems</li></ul> | Class A |
| | **For more information about these or any other drugs call the National Drugs Helpline on 0800 77 66 00** |

Table 3.4 *Continued*

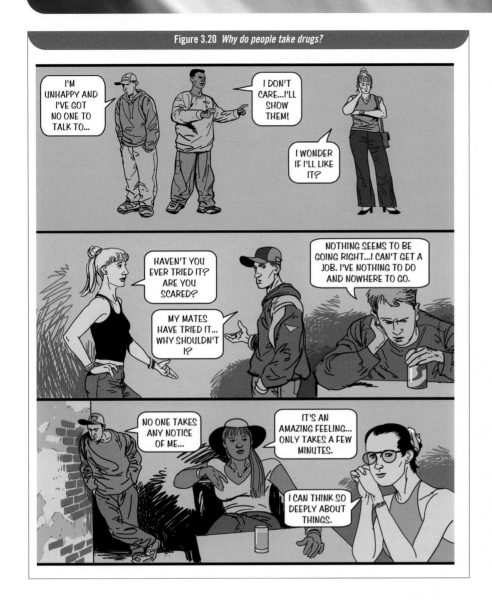

Figure 3.20 *Why do people take drugs?*

## Use and abuse of legal drugs

There are a number of drugs which are used legally. When their use is considered harmful or socially unacceptable, this is considered to be **abuse**. Far more deaths are caused each year through the abuse of legal drugs than from illegal drugs. The effects of excess alcohol intake and tobacco smoking are described below.

## Alcohol

*'I walked into the smoke-filled room and breathed a sigh of relief. It was obvious I could get what I was looking for: scoring is never very difficult in a place like this and it was obvious that I could not only get my drug of choice, but I could get it in any combination I desired. The dealers were polite enough, and even offered to bring it over to the table. I remembered the first time I had indulged. It used to make me sick, but over the years I had built up a tolerance.*

*Anyway, this was a drug I could handle; it made me feel better, more sociable; gave me a bit of a glow.'*

(An extract from *'Booze: Britain's real drug crisis'* in *The Independent*, 7.8.98.)

Reading the account above, you probably thought an illegal drug was being described, but this is an account of obtaining the legal drug, alcohol. However, just because a drug is legal it must not be considered harmless.

▶ There are an estimated 5000 deaths each year in England and Wales directly related to alcohol. (For heroine there are about 350 deaths in a year, and for ecstasy, fewer than 10.)

▶ Deaths from alcohol-related diseases have increased by more than a third in the past 10 years.

▶ One in 20 people are addicted to alcohol.

▶ About 27% of adult males drink above the level recommended by the medical profession.

▶ Alcohol costs the NHS £1.5 million a year.

▶ Alcohol costs British industry an estimated £2 billion a year due to absenteeism and poor performance.

▶ Alcohol is a factor in 40% of domestic violence.

Figure 3.21 shows the long-term effects of alcohol on the body.

### Young people and alcohol

▶ In 1997 1000 children under 15 were admitted to hospital suffering from acute alcohol poisoning.

▶ In the past 10 years 55 teenagers have died after drinking too much alcohol.

▶ Three-quarters of all 11 year olds have tried alcohol.

▶ The average weekly amount of alcohol consumed by 11–15 year olds doubled between 1990 and 1996.

▶ One thousand children aged under 15 are admitted to hospital each year with acute alcohol poisoning.

▶ Young people who regularly use alcohol are 22 times more likely to go on to use illegal drugs.

▶ Children of alcoholics have a greater risk of becoming alcoholics themselves.

What can parents do to help? The Health Education Authority give the advice to parents that they should not try to prevent children

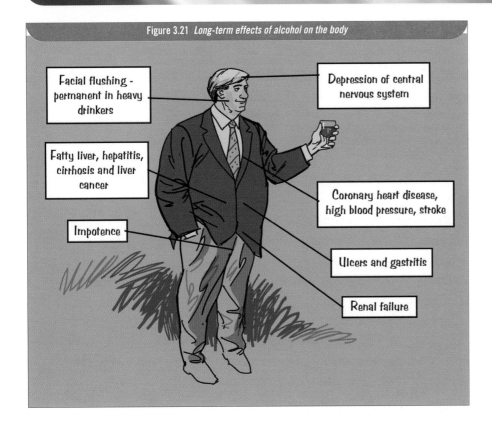

**Figure 3.21** *Long-term effects of alcohol on the body*

Facial flushing - permanent in heavy drinkers

Depression of central nervous system

Fatty liver, hepatitis, cirrhosis and liver cancer

Coronary heart disease, high blood pressure, stroke

Impotence

Ulcers and gastritis

Renal failure

from drinking and then drink too much themselves. They should talk about alcohol when the children are young and teach them that drinking in moderation is acceptable, but binge drinking can be very dangerous.

### Pregnancy and alcohol

Alcohol can stop the normal development of the foetus. Babies born to mothers who drink large amounts of alcohol throughout the pregnancy may be born with **foetal alcohol syndrome**. These children have facial deformities, stunted growth and mental retardation. More moderate drinking may increase the risk of miscarriage, but many women continue to drink small amounts of alcohol throughout their pregnancy with no ill effects. Pregnant women are recommended to have no more than one or two alcoholic drinks a week. The same advice is given to women who are breastfeeding.

### The elderly and alcohol

▶ At least a third of elderly drinkers did not have a problem with alcohol until they reached the age of 60.

▶ Older people are at greater risk of alcohol-related issues such as hypothermia, incontinence and depression.

▶ Elderly alcoholics suffer more severe withdrawal symptoms than younger people.

▶ Elderly people use the most prescription drugs, and alcohol can cause serious side effects when combined with many of these.

# Activity

1.  One of the most important things for drinkers to know is how the alcohol content of different drinks compare. Figure 3.22 shows drinks which contain roughly the same amount of alcohol. Each of these can be thought of as a **unit**. Figure 3.23 shows the limits people should keep below to avoid damaging their health.

    Copy out the table in Figure 3.24 to help you keep a diary of your alcohol consumption for a typical week (or, if more appropriate, ask an adult to do this for you). At the end of the week, calculate the number of units consumed. Compare this with the recommended limits. If the amount consumed is high, identify suitable opportunities for cutting down. (It is sometimes worth remembering **HALT**. This is to remind people that the occasions when there is the greatest temptation to drink too much are when someone is **hungry, angry, lonely** or **tired**.

2.  The following measures have been suggested to help limit the problems caused by excess drinking:

    ▶ the drink drive limits should be lowered
    ▶ more alcohol education should be provided for young people
    ▶ bottles and cans should be labelled with the number of units they contain
    ▶ better services should be provided to people addicted to alcohol.

    Discuss how useful you think each of these measures would be.

## Smoking

Smoking is the biggest single cause of preventable disease and premature death. There are five times more people killed by smoking than by road accidents, suicide, murder, AIDS and illegal drugs put together.

**Nicotine** is the powerful drug in tobacco which causes physical and psychological addiction to smoking. It increases heart rate and blood pressure.

**Tar** – this is black and sticky and contains cancer-causing chemicals (carcinogens). Tar clogs up the lungs and the chemicals are gradually absorbed, causing irritation and damage.

**Carbon monoxide** – this is a harmful gas which makes blood less efficient at carrying oxygen to the brain and muscles.

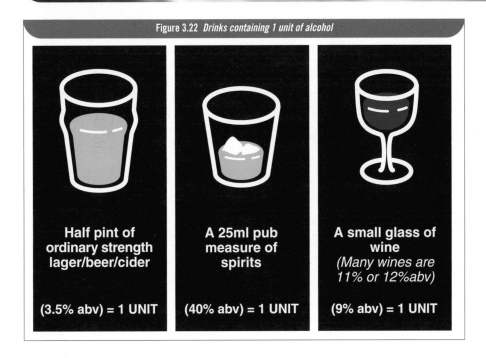

Figure 3.22 *Drinks containing 1 unit of alcohol*

**Half pint of ordinary strength lager/beer/cider**

**(3.5% abv) = 1 UNIT**

**A 25ml pub measure of spirits**

**(40% abv) = 1 UNIT**

**A small glass of wine**
*(Many wines are 11% or 12%abv)*

**(9% abv) = 1 UNIT**

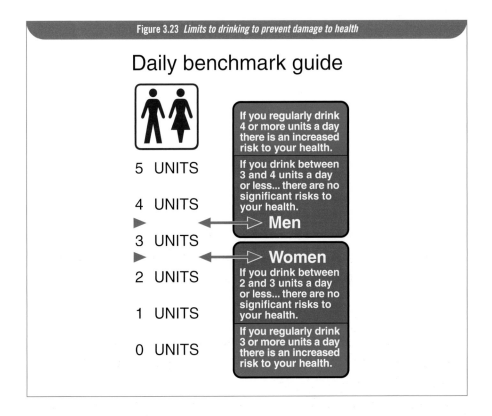

Figure 3.23 *Limits to drinking to prevent damage to health*

# Daily benchmark guide

5 UNITS

4 UNITS

3 UNITS

2 UNITS

1 UNITS

0 UNITS

If you regularly drink 4 or more units a day there is an increased risk to your health.

If you drink between 3 and 4 units a day or less... there are no significant risks to your health.

**Men**

**Women**

If you drink between 2 and 3 units a day or less... there are no significant risks to your health.

If you regularly drink 3 or more units a day there is an increased risk to your health.

Figure 3.24 *A drink diary*

## Drink Diary

|  | What? | Where / When / Who with? | Units |
|---|---|---|---|
| Mon |  |  |  |
| Tue |  |  |  |
| Wed |  |  |  |
| Thu |  |  |  |
| Fri |  |  |  |
| Sat |  |  |  |
| Sun |  |  |  |
|  |  | TOTAL |  |

The harmful effects of smoking are summarised in Figure 3.25.

### Young people and smoking

The longer someone smokes, the greater their chance of serious health problems later on. Because nicotine is addictive, the earlier someone starts smoking, the harder it is to give up in later life.

Trying out new things and taking risks is part of growing up, and figures show that 60% of all 15 year olds have smoked. Children are twice as likely to smoke if their parents are regular smokers.

### Pregnancy, parenthood and smoking

A pregnant woman who smokes is:

▶ more likely to have an underweight baby

▶ twice as likely to have a premature baby

▶ a third more likely to have a stillborn baby

▶ more likely to have a miscarriage.

Children who have a parent who smokes are:

▶ at a higher risk of cot death

▶ a third more likely to suffer from glue ear, which causes partial deafness

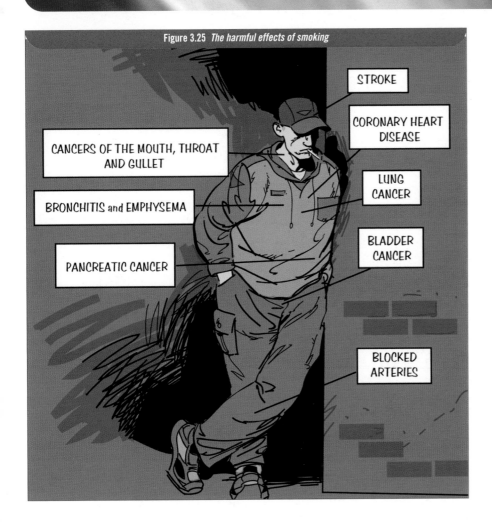

Figure 3.25 *The harmful effects of smoking*

▶ twice as likely to suffer from chest infections

▶ twice as likely to have asthma attacks.

17 000 under-fives are in hospital because of their parent's smoking.

It is, therefore, important that, as well as giving up smoking for the duration of the pregnancy, parents should make every effort not to smoke in the company of their young children.

### *The elderly and smoking*

Studies have shown that smokers aged 65 to 74 years old are almost 10 times more likely to die of lung cancer than those of this age group who do not smoke. Because of the harmful effects of continuing to smoke, even in old age, it is important that elderly people consider trying to stop. However, this may be more difficult for them because the longer a person has smoked for, the stronger the addiction to nicotine.

# Activity

1   Make a poster, leaflet or booklet aimed at encouraging a person to give up smoking. Aim it at either:

   ◗ a young person
   ◗ a pregnant woman
   ◗ a parent of a young child
   ◗ an elderly person.

2   Find out about the nicotine replacement therapies on offer – patches, gums and inhalers. How much do they cost, how are they used and, if you have the opportunity to talk to users, how successful are they?

## An unbalanced, poor quality or inadequate diet

If a person's diet is not balanced, and has an excess or inadequate amount of particular nutrients, their health will suffer. In developing countries the most common causes of malnutrition are lack of protein and energy in the diet, but in developed countries unhealthy diets tend to include too much salt, sugar, and fatty foods which are linked to cancer, heart disease, stroke and tooth decay.

### Obesity

Obesity or fatness runs in families and results from taking in more energy from the diet than is used up by the body. This is likely to happen if a person has a high sugar and/or fat diet.

Obesity can lead to emotional and social problems, as well as physical problems such as an increased likelihood of suffering from heart problems, high blood pressure, cancer of the colon and diabetes. It contributes to 30 000 deaths a year in the UK. A recent committee of MPs recently produced a report which says that by 2005 one in five men and one in four women may be obese. It recommended that, in order to reduce obesity:

   ◗ free fruit should be made available in schools

   ◗ there should be more cycle lanes

   ◗ children should have two hours' exercise a week in school

   ◗ GPs should improve the advice they give to patients about the dangers of obesity.

## Anorexia nervosa

Anorexia is often, but wrongly, known as the slimmer's disease. It mainly affects adolescent girls, although it can affect children from as young as seven to people in middle age, and males as well as females can be affected (Figure 3.26).

People with anorexia are likely to show the following characteristics:

▶ extreme weight loss

▶ overactivity and excessive exercising

▶ tiredness and weakness

▶ lanugo (baby-like hair on the body; thinning of hair on head)

▶ extreme choosiness over food.

There are various theories of what causes the illness. For example:

▶ those affected by anorexia see it as a way of taking control over their lives.

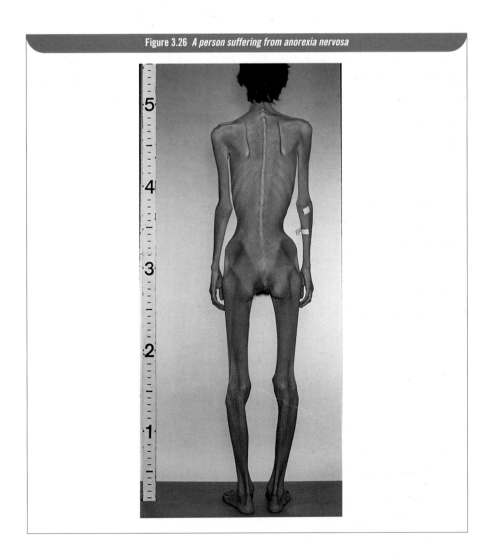

Figure 3.26 *A person suffering from anorexia nervosa*

> affected individuals do not wish to grow up and are trying to keep their childhood shape. This may result partly from the media obsession with achieving the 'perfect' (i.e. slim) body.

> it may be a physical illness caused partly by hormonal changes.

> it may be caused by depression.

### Bulimia nervosa

Bulimia nervosa is characterised by episodes of compulsive overeating, usually followed by self-induced vomiting. Again, the majority of individuals affected are female.

> The affected individual may be of normal weight, or only slightly underweight.

> Bingeing or vomiting may occur once or several times a day.

> The individual may have depression.

> The acid present in the vomit may damage the enamel of the teeth.

As with anorexia, there is no single cause to account for the disorder.

# Activity

1 (i) Collect photographs from magazines of models wearing clothes which are likely to appeal to young women. Do the models look healthy? Do you think that the body shape of these models is likely to influence adolescent girls?

(ii) *'Teenage dolls (such as Cindy and Barbie) promote an idealised role model which is unhealthy and can damage the self-concept of the child.'*

Discuss what this statement means, and whether you agree with it.

2 Read the newspaper article on salt (Figure 3.27) in the diet, and answer the following questions.
(i) List the diseases a high-salt diet is thought to cause.
(ii) In which foods is most of the salt in our diet found?
(iii) What is recommended as the maximum amount of salt we should have in our diet?
(iv) What does the food industry say we need salt for?

3 Look back at Tables 3.2 and 3.3 to check the deficiency diseases caused by the lack of vitamins and minerals.

**Figure 3.27** *An article from the Observer, 7 June 1997*

# Food giants want you to carry on eating salt – even if it kills you

### By Marie Woolf and John Illman

The food industry is fighting a rearguard action to keep Britons on a high-salt diet – although it can cause high blood pressure and lead to strokes, heart attacks and kidney failure.

High salt intake has been linked to stomach cancer and there is growing evidence that it could cause loss of calcium and be a major factor in osteoporosis (thinning of bones).

About 80 per cent of the salt Britons eat is hidden in processed foods, some of which contain as much salt as sea-water. The Committee of Medical Aspects of Food recently warned that we should eat no more than six grams of salt a day (about one level teaspoon), yet the average adult has nine grams.

The food industry claims salt is needed because it acts as a flavour enhancer, preservative and processing aid. The present government has to decide whether to bow to pressure from the industry or issue guidance on cutting down on salt. 'Salt should be the number one nutrition priority' said Jack Winkler, a food policy analyst.

## Too much stress

If there is a change in a person's life that they find difficult to cope with, we say they are suffering from stress.

If a person is under excessive stress, they will perform a task poorly. However, stress should not always be thought of as entirely negative. If a person is completely lacking stress, to the point at which they are bored, there will also be a decline in their ability to perform a task (Figure 3.28). This means that for each person there will be an optimum level of stress that will help them perform to the best of their ability.

Stress and how we manage our stress levels is linked directly to our health. A constant unmanageable level of stress will lead to physical, emotional and intellectual ill health.

When a person is under stress, the hormone adrenaline is produced. This hormone prepares you for what is known as the **alarm** or **fight or flight** reaction. Some of the effects of adrenaline include:

# Activity

1. Factors that cause stress are known as **stressors**. Examples of stressors are:
   ◗ bereavement
   ◗ the birth of a child
   ◗ moving house.
   Can you think of examples of other stressors?

2. Doctors sometimes classify people as Type A or Type B. Read the characteristics below and decide which type best describes you.

   | Characteristics of Type A: | Characteristics of Type B: |
   | --- | --- |
   | Hardworking | Easy-going manner |
   | A lot of drive | Relaxed |
   | Enjoy a challenge | Calm |
   | Feel guilty when relaxing | Non-aggressive |
   | Uneasy if not 'on the go' | Tolerant |
   | Competitive | |
   | Ambitious | |

   Type A people are more likely to suffer from stress. For example, they are twice as likely to develop coronary heart disease.

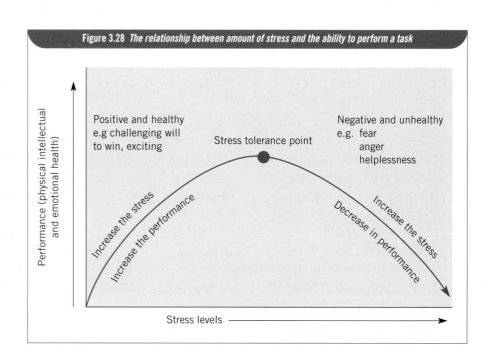

Figure 3.28 *The relationship between amount of stress and the ability to perform a task*

▶ an increased heart rate

▶ less blood flowing through the skin, which may make a person appear pale

▶ less blood flowing around the gut, which leads to the feeling of 'butterflies'

▶ increased sweating.

If the stress continues, eventually the adrenal gland, which produces adrenaline, will no longer function properly and the person will become ill. 270 000 British people are absent from work each day because of stress-related illnesses, and it is estimated that these cost £7 billion per year in sick pay, lost production and health service provision.

Stress has various effects on a person's health. For example:

▶ **physical health problems**, such as stomach ulcers, heart attacks, skin disorders such as eczema and psoriasis, myalgic encephalomyelitis (ME) (this used to be known, inaccurately, as yuppie flu)

▶ **emotional effects**, such as anxiety, insomnia and depression

▶ **behavioural effects**, such as increased smoking or consumption of alcohol.

Table 3.5 shows many of the short-term and long-term symptoms of stress.

| BEHAVIOURAL SHORT-TERM | PHYSICAL SHORT-TERM | EMOTIONAL SHORT-TERM |
|---|---|---|
| Overindulgence in smoking, alcohol or drugs | Headaches | Tiredness |
| Accidents | Back aches | Anixiety |
| Impulsive, emotional behaviour | Sleeping badly | Boredom |
| Poor relationships with others at home and at work | Indigestion | Irritability |
| Poor work performance | nausea | Depression |
| Emotional withdrawal | Dizziness | Inability to concentrate |
| | Excessive sweating | Apathy |
| | Trembling | |
| **BEHAVIOURAL LONG-TERM** | **PHYSICAL LONG-TERM** | **EMOTIONAL LONG-TERM** |
| Marital and family breakdown | Heart disease | Insomnia |
| Social isolation | Hypertension | Chronic depression and anxiety |
| | Ulcers | |
| | Poor general health | |

*Table 3.5 Symptoms of stress*

"Stress at Work" Health and Safety leaflet. Published by UNISON

Methods of coping with stressful situations may be either beneficial to a person's health or harmful to their health. For example, if you have an examination on a topic you find difficult, you may choose any of the following methods to help you cope, some of which are beneficial and some of which are harmful.

*Methods of coping which are beneficial to health*

▶ **Changing work patterns** – for example, you could draw up a revision timetable which allows you to spend an hour going through the work each evening with a friend.

▶ **Exercise** – for example, you could make time to go for an early morning swim.

▶ The use of **relaxation techniques** – for example, you could attend a yoga class.

▶ A **healthy diet** – you should make time to enjoy healthy, well-balanced meals.

▶ An **increase in leisure time** – for example, you could spend time at the weekend relaxing with friends.

▶ **Rest** – you should make sure you have at least 6–8 hours sleep a night.

*Methods of coping which are harmful to health*

▶ Increased use of tobacco, alcohol, tranquillisers, sleeping pills or illegal drugs.

▶ Long hours of studying causing lack of sleep.

# Activity

1. Interview a student to find out how they cope with stressful situations related to their studies, for example, important assignment deadlines or exams. Identify which of their methods of coping may be harmful to their health, and suggest more beneficial alternatives.

2. List the things that cause you stress. For example, waiting for a bus, sitting in a traffic jam, working on a difficult assignment, giving an oral presentation.

   Once you have identified the things that cause you stress, consciously try to relax in these situations and, where possible, do what you can to tackle the source of the problem. For example, before giving an oral presentation, make sure you are really well prepared, breathe in and then breathe out slowly a few times before starting, and consciously relax your shoulders.

# Lack of personal hygiene

A dictionary definition of hygiene (Figure 3.29) is *'The science concerned with the maintenance of health'*. However, we usually think of hygiene as being concerned with preventing pathogens entering the body. **Pathogens** are disease-causing organisms, mainly bacteria and viruses. These can enter the body through:

▶ the skin (for example, through cuts, sweat pores and hair follicles)

▶ the alimentary canal (gut)

▶ the respiratory tract (throat, trachea and lungs).

To maintain high levels of hygiene we need the following:

▶ efficient sewage disposal

▶ clean water supply

▶ efficient refuse disposal

▶ clean air (for example, good room ventilation)

▶ good personal hygiene (for example, care of teeth, hair and skin)

▶ safe food handling and preparation.

## Activity

Choose **one** of the six precautions necessary for good hygiene listed left, and prepare a poster to explain how it should be carried out. If you are working in a group, try to ensure that all six topics are covered.

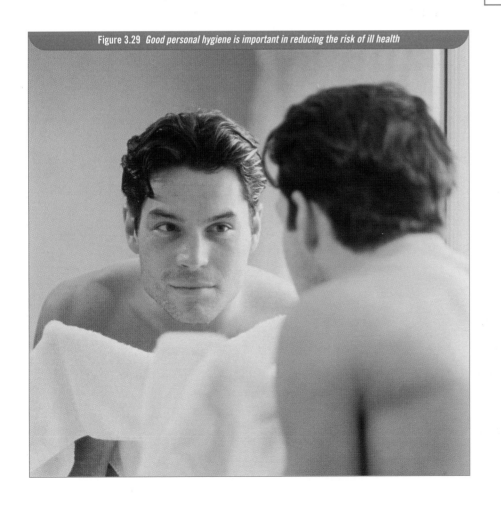

**Figure 3.29** *Good personal hygiene is important in reducing the risk of ill health*

# Lack of regular physical exercise

As the section on regular exercise (pages 212–213) explained, physical activity is important for all aspects of our health.

Evidence shows that by the age of 11 a third of all children are overweight, and a fifth of boys are obese. There is concern that lack of exercise in children will lead to problems for them in later life, for example, they will be at risk of developing heart disease and diabetes. Research has shown that the increased levels of obesity in children are not necessarily caused by diet. Today's children consume less fat and around 400 fewer calories than children in 1971. This suggests that the increased levels of obesity are caused by children today doing less exercise than children in the past. It is thought that the lack of exercise in children is the result of a number of different factors. These include:

▶ relying on cars instead of walking or cycling

▶ spending too much time in front of the television or computer (Figure 3.30 ) instead of playing outside

▶ a reduced number of games lessons at school.

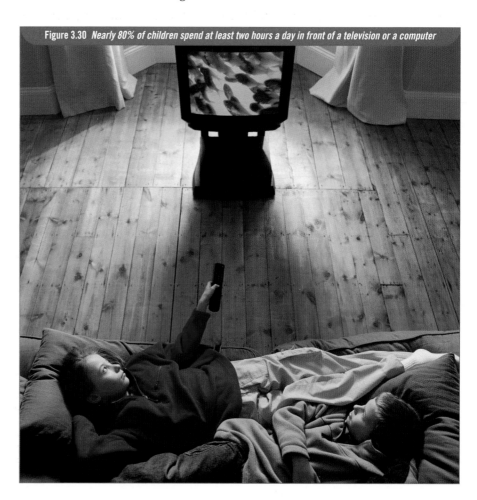

Figure 3.30 *Nearly 80% of children spend at least two hours a day in front of a television or a computer*

# Unprotected sex

In the 1980s in response to the discovery of AIDS, there were a number of prominent advertising campaigns alerting the public to the dangers of 'unsafe sex' (i.e. sexual intercourse without the use of a condom). As well as helping to control the spread of HIV, this also had the effect of limiting the number of cases of other sexually transmitted diseases (STDs). However, now people are apparently becoming more complacent about the need to practice safe sex, according to a recent survey. It found that the number of 18 to 20 year olds having unprotected sex had doubled in the past year. This helps to explains why the level of STDs is increasing again and why Britain has the highest teenage birth rate in Western Europe.

Look at Figure 3.31 for advice given by The Health Education Authority (now replaced by The Health Development Agency) on safer sex.

Table 3.6 lists some of the common STDs.

A person with an STD may have no symptoms, or they may have leakage from the penis or vagina, rashes, itchiness, sores, blisters, pain in the genital region, or a burning sensation when urinating or having sex. Most STDs can be treated quickly and easily, but some can cause long-term problems if untreated. It is, therefore, essential that anyone who is worried that they may have contracted an STD goes to the doctor or special clinic as soon as possible. The name of these clinics varies from one part of the country to another. It could be called Genito-Urinary Medicine (GUM) Clinic, Sexually Transmitted Disease Clinic, Venereal Disease (VD) Clinic, or Sexual Health Clinic. These treat everyone in confidence.

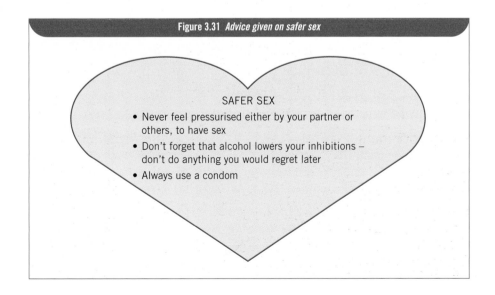

**Figure 3.31** *Advice given on safer sex*

SAFER SEX

- Never feel pressurised either by your partner or others, to have sex
- Don't forget that alcohol lowers your inhibitions – don't do anything you would regret later
- Always use a condom

Table 3.6 Some of the common STDs

**Genital herpes** (HSV) is caused by the herpes simplex virus. It can be passed on through skin contact with an infected person through kissing or sexual intercourse. It can affect the mouth, the genital area, the skin around the anus and the fingers in the form of blisters and sores, sometimes accompanied by flu-like symptoms. After the initial outbreak is over the virus hides away in the nerve fibres, where it remains totally undetected and causes no symptoms. It can recur when the person is ill or run down, but it is not severe in its symptoms. Treatment is usually unnecessary but tablets are available to reduce the severity of symptoms when it is first caught, if treated quickly.

**Gonorroea** is a bacterial infection. It is sexually transmitted and can infect the cervix, urethra, rectum, anus and throat. It sometimes causes no symptoms but can include discharge from the penis in men and vagina in women (including pain when urinating), and from the anus in both sexes. Treatment is administered through antibiotics. It is important for both sexes to receive treatment but women should be aware that it can lead to infertility if left untreated.

**Chlamydia** is the most common treatable bacterial sexually transmitted infection. It infects the cervix in women, and can infect the urethra, rectum and eyes in both sexes, causing discharge from the genitals, pain when passing urine, swollen eyes and other symptoms. Women should be checked if their sexual partner displays these symptoms, even if they expreience no symptoms themselves, as it can lead to infertility. Treatment is administered through antibiotics.

**Genital warts** are small fleshy growths which may appear anywhere on a man or woman's genital area. The are caused by the human papilloma virus (HPV) and are passed on through genital contact. They are treated by liquid solutions, by freezing or by lazers, but may need prolonged treatment before they disappear. It is also possible that they will recur so further check ups at a clinic of genito-urinary medicine (GUM) will be necessary. Treatment is important as some types of the wart may be linked to changes in the cervical cells which can lead to cervical cancer in women.

**HIV** (Human Immunodeficiency Virus) is a virus that can damage the body's defence system so that it cannot fight off certain infections. If someone with HIV goes on to get certain serious illnesses, this condition is called AIDS. The virus is passed on through unprotected sex with someone who has HIV, by sharing needles, syringes or other drug-injecting equipment with someone who has HIV, or from a mother with HIV to her baby during pregnancy, at birth or during breastfeeding. There are no early warning symptoms of the virus and at present there is no cure or vaccine. There are, however, new drugs that can control the level of HIV in the blood and delay the development of AIDS. HIV can be avoided by practising safe sex (any sex that does not allow blood, semen or fluid from the vagina to be exchanged internally, e.g. get inside the body) and by avoiding the sharing of needles when injecting drugs.

# Social isolation

People are considered to be socially isolated when they have low levels of social contact. They may find themselves in this situation for a variety of different reasons, for example, because of **poverty**, **homelessness** or **disability**. If a person is unhappy with their lack of contact with others, social isolation leads to feelings of loneliness. Those who are socially isolated complain of feelings of:

▶ abandonment

▶ unexplained dread

▶ time passing slowly

▶ inability to concentrate and make decisions

▶ feelings of uselessness

▶ doubts about their ability to survive.

# Activity

Have a go at the following quiz. (Answers on page 273).

1. Sexually transmitted diseases can cause:
   a) itchiness and a burning sensation when urinating
   b) infertility if untreated
   c) no symptoms
   d) all of the above.
2. To be effective, emergency contraceptive pills must be taken:
   a) the morning after having unprotected sex
   b) up to three days after having unprotected sex
   c) up to a week after having unprotected sex.
3. HIV can be passed by which of the following:
   a) kissing
   b) toilet seats
   c) towels
   d) sheets
   e) cups
   f) swimming pools
   g) unprotected sex.

Physical health can also be threatened by social isolation. A socially isolated person would be more likely to suffer from **hypothermia** (a dangerously low body temperature), for example.

Social isolation is often considered a particular problem for **elderly people**. This may be because:

▶ older people may outlive relatives and friends

▶ they are more likely to live alone

▶ disabilities and increased chronic illness may limit their mobility

▶ they may be unaware of available resources in their communities

▶ their social activities may be limited by poverty.

When working with people suffering from social isolation, health and social care professionals will encourage clients to talk about their feelings and try to help to identify and reduce factors that cause or contribute to their social isolation.

# Activity

Go to your local library or civic centre to find leaflets giving information on education, sporting and leisure activities, and volunteering opportunities for the elderly. Make posters to show what is available, and to encourage people to take advantage of what is on offer. If possible display these posters in a public place where they will be seen by people in this age group.

# Poverty

There is a strong link between poverty and health, for example:

▶ in 1999 the death rate from heart disease in the most deprived 20% of health authorities in England, was 26% higher than the national average

▶ in Newham (an area with high levels of poverty) people under 65 are 70% more likely to die of a heart attack or stroke than in England as a whole

▶ girls from the poorest backgrounds are 10 times more likely to become teenage mothers than those from the richest, and the infant mortality rates of babies born to teenage mothers is more than 50% higher than the average.

There are a number of problems associated with poverty that adversely affect health. A person's income will affect their diet, environment, education and housing. Smoking is more common amongst people in lower income groups and there are fewer primary care facilities available (for example, GP surgeries).

The **government poverty audit** includes people in households where the entire family income is less than half the national average household income. This is currently 12 million people, or 24% of the population. (This has risen from 5 million people in 1979.)

▶ A single adult is considered to be living in poverty if s/he has an income of less than £73.50 per week (after housing costs).

▶ A couple with no children is considered to be living in poverty if they have an income of less than £133.50 per week (after housing costs).

▶ Two adults with three children are considered to be living in poverty if they have an income of less than £223 per week (after housing costs).

Certain groups face especially high risks of poverty. In the UK a third of children, half of lone-parent families, about 40% of pensioners, and about 70% of families where the breadwinner is unemployed live in poverty.

There is evidence to show that it is not just poverty that has a harmful effect on health. **Relative poverty** means being poor in a rich society, and it is thought that this has the worst effect on health. Societies with small differences between incomes have lower death rates than societies with large differences between incomes. It is, therefore, worrying that in the UK the gap between the people with the lowest incomes (mainly pensioners, children and women) and the people with the highest incomes is growing.

▶ The poorest 10% of the population have incomes no higher than they did virtually two decades ago.

▶ Over the same period the income of the richest 10% grew by one half.

▶ The gap between those with middle incomes and both higher and lower incomes has also grown.

# Inadequate housing

It is difficult to know to what extent poor housing affects health. This is because people who live in unhealthy homes usually suffer from other forms of disadvantage, such as poor diet, unemployment or poor education. A report by the Royal Institution of Chartered Surveyors concluded that thousands of people are killed every year by poor housing. Most of the 1.5 million homes that are officially classed as 'unfit for human habitation' are occupied. Poor housing is not only a problem in urban areas. In rural areas wages are low, and high unemployment means that it can be difficult for young people to afford accommodation.

## Activity

1. In 1999 a minimum wage was introduced by the government. Find out the current minimum wage, and then in a group discuss the following.
   ▶ Has the minimum wage been set at a reasonable level?
   ▶ What are the advantages and disadvantages of setting a minimum wage?
   (Answers on page 273).
2. Read the following quote and then discuss whether you agree with it and, if so, why.

*"The way to reduce ill health in impoverished areas is to reduce poverty. The most important steps any government can take are to increase the incomes of those on income support, to increase child benefit, to guarantee high quality pre-school education, and to reduce real rents in housing. Social expenditure is likely to have more effect in the long-term than health expenditure."*

*Characteristics of poor housing that have a direct effect on health*

▶ **Faulty design** may contribute to fires and falls in the home. Most house fires occur in poor and inadequate housing. Children from the lowest social class are 16 times more likely to die in a house fire than people from the highest social class.

▶ **Inadequate lighting** can be linked to falls.

▶ **Damp** is related to the growth of moulds and mites, and thus linked to respiratory diseases such as asthma. It is estimated that over 2.5 million homes in the UK suffer from severe dampness.

▶ **Inadequate heating** may lead to hypothermia, particularly in the elderly. The poorest usually live in badly insulated homes which are the most expensive to heat.

▶ **Poor sanitation**, for example, the shared washing facilities in bedsits and bed-and-breakfast hostels, can lead to the spread of disease.

▶ **Inadequate food storage and cooking facilities** increase the incidence of food poisoning and make a poor diet more likely.

# Activity

1. Read the following account of a young mother's living conditions. Write a list of the health problems she and her young child have, and for each suggest how these may have been caused by aspects of their housing. (See page 274 for answers.)

> Sally lives with her child, Sam, in bed-and-breakfast accommodation. They have one room and share a kitchen, toilet and bathroom with two other families. Their room is on the second floor which makes life difficult as Sam is still in a pushchair. In their room there is a problem with damp in the winter, and this is made worse because Sally has to dry their clothes on a radiator. There are no nearby shops, so she often has to rely on fish and chips from the mobile food van that visits. When she leaves food in the shared fridge it often disappears, so she keeps most of their food in the bottom of her wardrobe. Sally gets fed up with all the rules: children aren't allowed to play in the corridor; there is no hot water after 10pm; the kitchen is locked at 9pm; no visitors are allowed. Since they have lived there, Sam has suffered from asthma, Sally occasionally has a bad back, and they both sometimes have diarrhoea. Recently Sally has been feeling depressed.

2. There is a high incidence of mental illness amongst homeless people. Discuss whether you think mental illness leads to homelessness, or whether homelessness leads to mental health problems.

# Unemployment

Ill health can result from the stress and/or poverty caused by:

▶ unemployment

▶ job insecurity (the threat of being made unemployed)

▶ low wages.

There is a lot of evidence to show that people in employment have better health and well-being than those who are unemployed. The following have all been found to be higher amongst the unemployed:

▶ death rates

▶ amount of long-term illness

▶ disability

▶ psychological illness

▶ risk of suicide

▶ stomach ulcers.

# Environmental pollution

Pollution of the environment can have a significant effect on our health and well-being.

## Water pollution

Humans need water for a variety of uses. It must be clear and not contaminated with pollutants, in order to prevent infectious diseases and poisoning. Toxic chemicals, industrial, agricultural and domestic waste are common pollutants of water. Purification is carried out on water before it is used, but although the treatment can remove organic waste and some bacterial contamination, it cannot cope with heavy chemical pollution. Examples of chemical pollutants in water include the following:

▶ **Lead** – this is taken into the body via food, air and water. It concentrates in the liver, kidneys and bones. There is evidence that it can cause mental retardation in children.

▶ **Nitrates** enter water from fertilisers which are leached out of soil.

## Air pollution

Children are particularly susceptible to air pollution, partly because of their large lung surface area to body volume ratio, which is a factor of their small size.

Asthma is a condition thought largely to result from air pollution, particularly from traffic emissions.

*Some asthma facts*

▶ Asthma affects one in seven children.

▶ It is the most important cause of emergency hospital admissions.

▶ Respiratory diseases account for a third of children's GP visits.

▶ Asthma accounts for one in 20 childhood deaths.

▶ Hospital admissions for asthma have increased 13-fold since the early 1960s.

**Lead** is the most serious heavy-metal pollutant in the atmosphere. The lead in car exhaust fumes accounts for 80%, with the remainder coming from industrial processes. Even very low levels of lead in the blood can affect cognitive development and behaviour, and growth can be affected.

Traffic is predicted to rise by 87% over the next 30 years. While vehicles are producing fewer harmful emissions there are more of them and people will travel longer distances.

## Noise pollution

Noise is defined as unwanted sound. Because it can be a health hazard, it is considered as a form of pollution. Noise maps produced by the Council for the Protection of Rural England show that there are very few tranquil areas remaining in England. With forecasts of huge traffic increases in the next twenty years, noise levels are set to increase further.

Sounds above 90 dB (decibels) can damage hearing. If exposure is over a long period, this damage can be permanent.

# Activity

1.  One way to cut down on the air pollution is to reduce our use of cars.
    **(i)** Can you think of ways in which you or your family could reduce your number of car journeys?
    **(ii)** Can you think of ways of encouraging other people to reduce their dependence on cars?

2.  You can find out about air pollution levels in your area from your local authority health department. Air quality is also monitored nationally, and in *Resources* on page 269 there are details of where you can find this information.

# INDICATORS OF PHYSICAL HEALTH

Some indicators of physical health can be measured. Examples include:

▶ blood pressure

▶ peak flow

▶ body mass index

▶ resting pulse and recovery after exercise.

## Blood pressure

The pressure at which blood flows through the circulatory system can be used as an indicator of health. It is measured using a **sphygmomanometer** (or **sphygmo** for short.) Traditionally a mercury column sphygmomanometer has been used for measuring blood pressure. However, there are a number of drawbacks associated with these:

▶ European legislation requires the phasing out of all equipment containing mercury

▶ using such models is a skilled operation requiring the use of a stethoscope

▶ there are no audible or visual indicators of pressure measurements for a group of people (for example, in a classroom situation) to experience.

There are, therefore, advantages in using an electronic model (Figure 3.32). A cuff is inflated around the upper arm. The high pressure compresses the brachial artery which has the effect of stopping the blood flow to the lower arm. The cuff is then slowly deflated and as the blood flow resumes, the sounds are detected by the microphone that is built into the cuff. Measurements are read from a gauge or digital display. Some models provide a reading of pulse as well (see page 260).

Blood pressure is recorded as two numbers – the **systolic** over **diastolic** pressure.

▶ The **systolic pressure** is the pressure when the heart is contracting and is therefore the higher value.

▶ The **diastolic pressure** is the pressure when the heart is relaxing and is therefore the lower value.

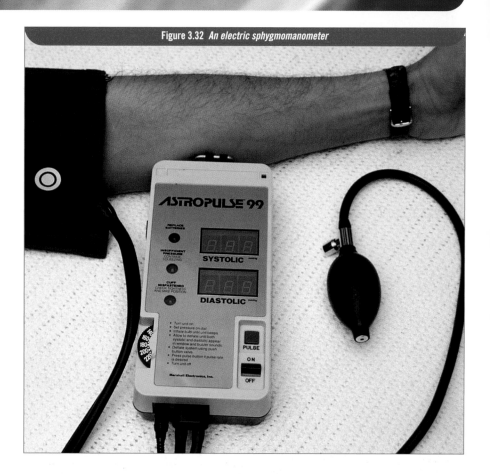

Figure 3.32 *An electric sphygmomanometer*

120/80 mmHg is a normal reading. This increases with age.

▶ A person who suffers from **hypotension** has a **low blood pressure**.

▶ A person who suffers from **hypertension** has a **high blood pressure**. A blood pressure of more than 140 systolic and 90 diastolic is considered abnormal.

## Peak flow

Peak flow is a measure of how fast you can blow air out of your lungs. It can be measured with a **peak flow meter** (Fig. 3.33). When you blow into a peak flow meter it measures the speed of air passing through the meter. This figure is given in cubic decimetres ($dm^3$, i.e. litres) per minute. Peak flow readings vary according to sex, age, height and even the time of day the measurement is taken.

▶ Peak flow readings are usually higher in men than women.

▶ The highest peak flow usually occurs between the ages of 30 to 40 years.

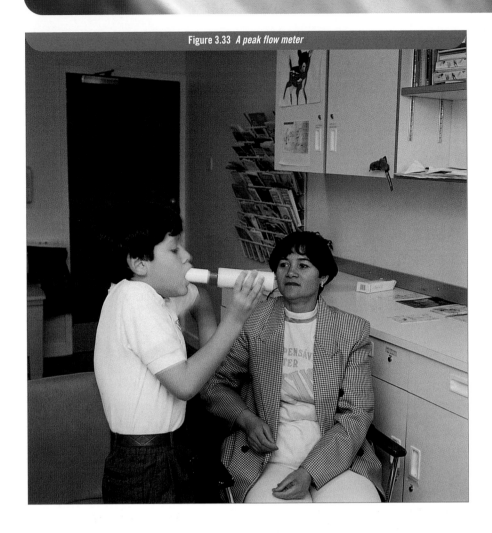

Figure 3.33 *A peak flow meter*

▶ The taller a person is, the higher their peak flow is likely to be.

▶ Peak flow is often higher in the morning than in the evening.

Peak flow measurements are often used to diagnose and monitor the severity of **asthma**. People with asthma have narrowed airways taking air to the lungs. This may be because the linings of the airways are swollen, or because there is mucus in the airways, or because the tubes are constricted by the muscles surrounding the airways. All of these reduce the amount of air that can flow through the airways. This means that asthma sufferers will have a low peak flow reading, and the more severe their asthma, the lower their reading. Asthma sufferers will have a peak flow reading of 200–400 dm$^3$/min., compared with a normal value of 400–600 dm$^3$/min. Because peak flow may vary tremendously from time to time, a one-off reading at a surgery may not give a doctor or nurse sufficient information. The asthma sufferer will, therefore, be asked to take their own readings morning and evening over a period of time and plot them on a chart (Figure 3.34).

**Figure 3.34** *Peak flow charts*

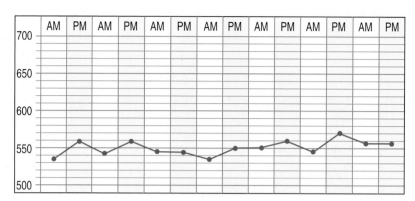

1.Peak flow chart of a person without asthma or a person whose asthma is well controlled

**Figure 3.35** *Axes for plotting your scattergram*

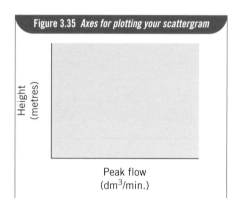

Height (metres)

Peak flow (dm³/min.)

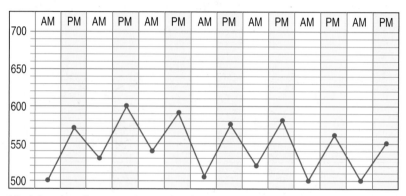

1.Peak flow chart of a person whose asthma is not well controlled

# Activity

If you have access to a peak flow meter, carry out an investigation into how height affects peak flow.

i)  First write down a **hypothesis** (in other words, a guess at what your results will show).

ii)  Collect measurements of height and peak flow from at least ten people. (Remember to try to keep other variables constant. For example, take measurements from people who are the same age and the same sex.) Put your results into a table.

iii)  Plot a **scattergram** using axes for your graph, as shown in Figure 3.35. (Each person's height and peak flow reading will be plotted as a single point, so you will end up with the same number of points as people measured.)

iv)  Are the points arranged randomly, or can you find a **line of best fit**? If you can, this suggests that there is a **correlation** between height and peak flow.

v)  If height and peak flow tend to increase together, we say there is a **positive** correlation. However, if as height increases, peak flow tends to decrease, we say there is a **negative** correlation. If your results show a correlation, is it a positive or negative correlation?

vi)  Look back at your hypothesis. Do your results support your hypothesis or not?

# Body Mass Index (BMI)

A person's **weight** can be an important guide to their physical health. If someone is very overweight or underweight it is obviously cause for concern about their physical health. However, as the example on the right shows, a measurement of weight alone will not give sufficient information to allow conclusions to be reached about physical fitness.

To allow any conclusions to be drawn about physical health from the weight of a person, we obviously need to have an idea of their **height** too. In the example above, you would have formed a different opinion of Paul's physical health if you had been told that he was 1.83 m or 1.60 m. Height should be measured as shown in Figure 3.36.

## Activity

Paul is an 18-year-old student who weighs 77 kg. Can you make any comments on the state of his physical health?

What other piece of information would be most useful to help you form an opinion?

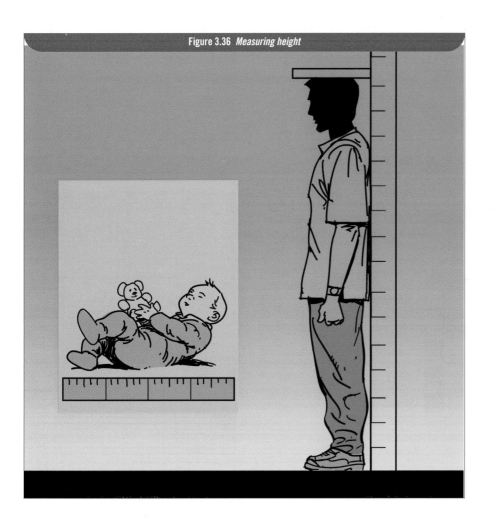

**Figure 3.36** *Measuring height*

# Activity

Figure 3.37 shows the relationship between weights and heights.

1.  Take a straight line across from your height and a line up from your weight.
    (When you weigh yourself, take 2 kg off to allow for your clothes.) Check which category you fit into. Does this mean you need to alter your diet/exercise regime? If so, how?

2.  Looking at Figure 3.37, what advice would you give to the following people about their diet/exercise based on their weights and heights?
    ▶ Palin: 65 kg/1.55 m
    ▶ Kate: 47 kg/1.68 m
    ▶ Peter: 70 kg/1.75 m
    (See page 274 for answers.)

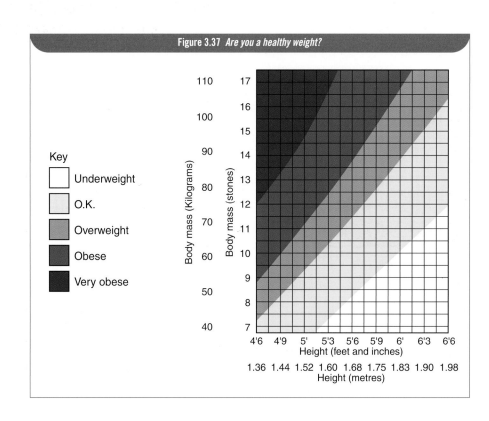

Figure 3.37 *Are you a healthy weight?*

Key

☐ Underweight
☐ O.K.
☐ Overweight
☐ Obese
☐ Very obese

Body mass (Kilograms)
Body mass (stones)

Height (feet and inches)
Height (metres)

Body mass index is a measure that takes into account both height and weight. It can, therefore, be used to indicate whether a person's weight is healthy for their height.

Body mass index (BMI) is given by the equation:

$$BMI = \frac{Mass\ (kg)}{(Height/m)^2}$$

This means that to calculate your BMI you should:

i) Use your calculator to find the square of your height in metres (for example, a height of 1.63 m will have a squared value of $1.63 \times 1.63 = 2.82 m^2$).

ii) Divide your mass in kg by the value calculated in step (i). This gives you your BMI.

iii) Compare your calculated BMI with the values given below:

| Body mass index | Interpretation |
|---|---|
| Below 20 | Underweight |
| 20–25 | Ideal weight |
| 25.1–30 | Overweight |
| Above 30 | Obese |

Note: Research projects which would involve asking people their weights should be avoided, as some may feel very uncomfortable giving this information.

## Activity

1. Table 3.7 shows the height and weight of three 18-year-old students. For each of them calculate their BMI and say which of them are overweight.
   (See page 274 for answers)

2. Read the article from *The Times* (27/4/99).
   What would be:
   i) the main advantage and
   ii) the main disadvantage
   of using waist measurement to diagnose obesity?
   (See page 274 for answers).

Table 3.7 *Height and mass of three eighteen-year-old students*

|  | Height (m) | Mass (kg) |
|---|---|---|
| Guy | 1.60 | 74 |
| Heather | 1.50 | 54 |
| Rachel | 1.75 | 77 |

Figure 3.38 *An article from The Times, 27/4/99*

### How to tape obesity's measure

People who worry about their weight have made a trip to the bathroom scales the second most urgent task each morning. There is now a simpler regime and a tape measure is all that is needed.

Once the girth of the waist is known doctors should have an immediate idea whether they are dealing with a problem of obesity and, if so, how bad it is.

It has now been shown that a simple waist measurment is all that is needed to assess obesity. Women should have a waist measurement of not more than 32in (80cm) and men 37in (94cm). As long as they keep within these parameters, they don't have to worry too much about having pudding. Doctors will start to get concerned about a female patient if her waist measurement reaches 35in (88cm) or a man has a waistband of 40in (102cm) or above.

Doctors good at mental arithmatic still like to work out the BMI (the body mass index), which is calculated by dividing the patient's weight in kilograms by his or her height in metres squared. If the BMI is more than 25, the patient has exceeded the recommended calculation and is considered overweight, if more than 30, he or she is technically obese and if the figure is more than 40, grossly obese.

# Resting pulse rate and recovery after exercise

The pumping action of the heart causes a regular pulsation in the blood flow. This can be felt by pressing two finger tips against either the wrist just below the base of the thumb (Figure 3.39) or on the neck a few centimetres below the jaw. It is often most convenient to count for 15 seconds and multiply by four to calculate the number of beats per minute. The pulse rate corresponds to the heart rate, which varies according to the person's state of relaxation or physical activity.

## Resting pulse rate

The resting pulse rate is the pulse rate taken after a period of relaxation. It should be taken at least three times and an average (mean) calculated. A low resting pulse rate generally indicates a better physical fitness level than a person with a higher resting pulse rate.

▶ In reasonably fit individuals their pulse rate will be between 60 and 80 beats per minute, and on average 72 beats per minute in adults.

Figure 3.39 *How to locate the pulse at the wrist*

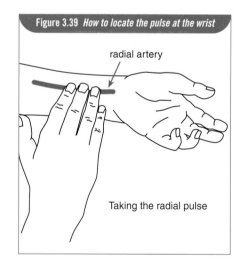

radial artery

Taking the radial pulse

- In children and the elderly it will be higher than in young adults.
- Men, on average, have lower pulse rates than women.
- In top distance athletes it could be as low as 40 beats per minute.

# Activity

**i)** Take the resting pulse rate of at least three people who regularly take exercise (for example, people who compete regularly in a sport) and three people who take very little exercise. Allow each person at least five minutes of relaxation before counting their pulse. Count for 15 seconds and multiply by four to give you pulse rate in beats per minute. Don't forget to make three counts of each person's pulse and calculate their mean pulse rate:

$$\text{(mean pulse rate} = \frac{\text{pulse rate 1} + \text{pulse rate 2} + \text{pulse rate 3}}{3}\text{)}$$

**ii)** Plot a bar graph to show the mean pulse rate of each person. Shade the bars to distinguish between the pulse rates of people who exercise and the pulse rates of those who do not.

**iii)** Do your results show lower resting pulse rates in the people who take more exercise? If not, suggest reasons for any unexpected results. For example, it is difficult to measure the amount of exercise people take; there are many factors other than exercise that affect fitness.

## Recovery after exercise

Another way of using pulse rate as an indicator of the level of a person's physical fitness is to see how quickly after a period of exercise a person recovers and gets back to their own normal pulse rate.

A **fitness index** can be calculated to measure a person's ability to recover after exercise.

**Equipment**: step/bench/or box 50 cm high; stop watch; metronome or tape with two-second bleeps.

**Procedure**: if possible, work in pairs. Step up and down on the step, as shown in Figure 3.40, at the rate of 30 steps per minute (one step should take two seconds). Ask your partner to check that you are stepping at the correct rate. If you can, keep on stepping for four minutes. If you find this too much, stop, sit down, and your partner should write down how many seconds you have managed (out of a total of 240). Rest in a sitting position for 60 seconds. Your partner should then take your pulse for 30 seconds

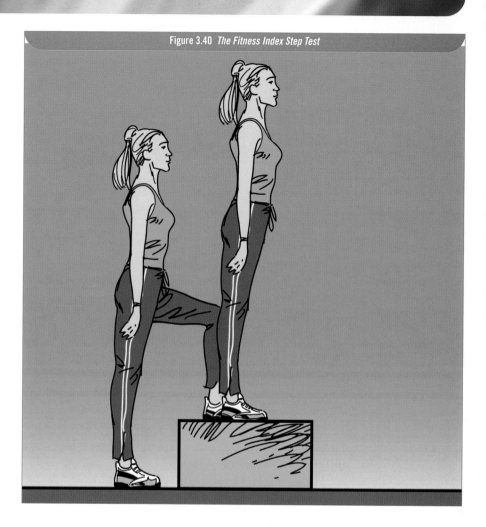

Figure 3.40 *The Fitness Index Step Test*

while you remain sitting and then write down the number of beats. Continue resting for a further 30 seconds, and then have your pulse taken again for 30 seconds. Write down the number of beats. Sit for another 30 seconds and then have your pulse counted for a final 30 seconds. Write down the number of beats. (By now you will have had your pulse taken for thirty seconds one, two and three minutes after finishing exercise.)

Calculations:

Time of exercise = 4 minutes = 240 seconds (or less if you had to stop earlier)

Total number of pulse counts = pulse count 1 + pulse count 2 + pulse count 3

(For example: 80 + 70 + 60)

$$\text{Score} = \frac{\text{time of exercise in seconds} \times 100}{\text{total pulse counts} \times 2}$$

For example:

$$240 \times 100$$
$$(80 + 70 + 60) \times 2$$

Compare your score with those shown in Table 3.8.

| FITNESS INDEX SCORE | RATING |
|---|---|
| 90 and over | Excellent |
| 80–89 | Good |
| 65–79 | Fair |
| 55–64 | Poor |
| 54 and below | Very poor |

*Table 3.8 Fitness Index scores*

# Activity

1. Measure the fitness index of two volunteers, preferably of the same sex and the same age. Can you explain the results you find? For example, does the person with the higher score do more exercise or have a healthier diet than the person with the lower score?

2. Take your resting pulse rate twice and record the lowest score. Do five minutes of step exercise as explained above. After completing the exercise wait for one minute and then take your pulse rate. (Take it for 30 seconds and then multiply by two to give you pulse rate in beats per minute.) Continue taking your pulse rate at intervals of one minute until your pulse rate returns to normal. Plot the recovery to the resting rate on a graph (i.e. plot pulse rate against time on a line graph. In a different colour on the same graph draw a straight line to show your resting pulse rate).

   ▶ How many minutes does it take for your pulse rate to return to the resting rate?

   ▶ Find the ratio of your resting pulse rate relative to your pulse rate after exercise (e.g. 70 beats per minute at rest relative to 140 beats per minute after exercise, gives a ratio of 70:140, or 1:2).

# HEALTH PROMOTION AND IMPROVEMENT METHODS

There are a number of different definitions of health promotion, but one which is often used is the WHO (World Health Organisation) definition:

*Health promotion is the process of enabling people to increase control over, and to improve, their health.*

Health promotion involves providing information to others which will help them to improve their health and well-being. It may also include the development of **health improvement plans**, either for groups or individuals.

## Stages in the development of a health improvement plan

1. The **health risks** of a person, or group, must be identified from:

   ▶ **physical health assessment**, for example, measuring blood pressure, body mass index or pulse rate at rest and after exercise (see *Indicators of physical health* on page 253).

   ▶ **lifestyle information**.

2. **Targets** must be set. What health improvements are we aiming for?

3. **Methods** and **activities** must be planned. What **health behaviours** will bring about the hoped for health improvements?

4. **Resources** must be identified. What health promotion materials are available to inform, motivate and support people to improve their health and well-being? For example, which organisations, books, leaflets, posters, advertisements and websites will provide useful health promotion materials? (See *Resources* on page 269.)

5. The health improvement plan is **implemented**.

6. The success of the health plan must be **evaluated**. Have the targets been met? If not, why not? What improvements could be made?

## Some of the features of a successful health plan

▶ As much information as possible must be gathered on **lifestyle** and **physical indicators of good health** to allow the risks of an individual or a group to be identified.

- The plan should consider **physical**, **social** and **emotional** health.

- The person putting the plan together has **empathy** for the feelings of the person for whom the plan has been created, and understands that a person's choice about their health and well-being can be affected by self-esteem, financial factors and social pressures.

- The plan should include **short-** and **long-term targets** with **time scales**. For example, a short-term target could be to increase physical activity which in the long-term would improve levels of fitness.

- Targets should be **realistic**. For example, a very rapid weight loss may be considered unrealistic.

- The **strengths** and **weaknesses** of the plan should be identified. It is important to remember that activities to improve health, such as dieting and increasing exercise, involve determination from the person following the plan. It is likely that some parts of the plan will be more challenging to achieve than other parts and these should be anticipated with suggestions made of how to overcome difficulties.

- The plan, including the language used, should **reflect the needs and abilities of the chosen target**, for example, child, adolescent, adult or elderly person.

- Relevant **health promotional material** should be identified and used appropriately. (See *Resources* on page 269.)

## Activity

1. The website www.HealthCentral.com allows you to create a health profile by answering a number of questions on your lifestyle. It then identifies your greatest health risks and gives you advice on changes you could make to improve your health. Have a go!

2. Produce a health improvement plan for an individual. Choose a person from one of the case studies below.

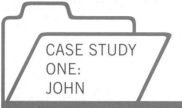

CASE STUDY
ONE:
JOHN

**Lifestyle information**

John is 52. Three years ago he was made redundant from his job working in a factory. Now he works in a pub five nights a week. He is usually cheerful and enjoys a good social life at work. He is divorced and lives alone. He will sometimes fry himself some food, but generally he snacks at home and relies on pub food, such as pie and chips, in the evening. He smokes about twenty cigarettes a day and usually drinks about five pints of beer a day. He walks a short distance to the bus stop where he catches a bus to work, which is about a mile from where he lives, but does very little other exercise.

**Measures of health**

The following measurements were recorded for John at a recent physical examination:

Height:              1.75 m
Weight:              102 kg
Peak flow:           510 dm$^3$/min
Resting pulse rate:  88 beats per min
Pulse rate after four minute of exercise:
Time (min) after exercise:   Pulse rate (beats per 30 seconds):
1  85
2  76
3  67
Other observations: John's father died from a heart attack, and his brother suffers from heart trouble.

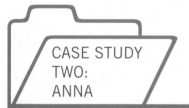

CASE STUDY
TWO:
ANNA

**Lifestyle information**

Anna is a 25-year-old accountant. She has a good income and has recently bought a flat where she lives alone. She finds her work stressful. Because she works such long hours and is exhausted when she gets home, she complains that her social life is non-existent. She is too tired to cook when she gets in, and tends to have a quick glass of wine and snack in front of the TV before falling into bed. At weekends she spends most of her time revising for accountancy exams.

## Measures of health

The following measurements were recorded for Anna at a recent physical examination:

Height:              1.60 m
Weight:              42 kg
Peak flow:           475 dm³/min
Resting pulse rate:  82 beats per min
Pulse rate after four minutes of exercise:
Time (min) after exercise:   Pulse rate (beats per 30 seconds):
1  78
2  60
3  48

Other observations: Anna complains of usually feeling tense and finding it difficult to relax.

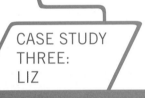

## CASE STUDY THREE: LIZ

## Lifestyle information

Liz is a 17-year-old Health and Social Care student. In the week she is at college and spends most evenings either doing course work or working on the checkout in a local supermarket. At weekends she relaxes by going out with her friends, either to parties or local nightclubs. Although she does not drink during the week, she often drinks heavily at the weekends and sometimes cannot remember incidents from the night before. She sometimes uses cannabis.

## Measures of health

The following measurements were recorded for Liz at a recent physical examination:

Height:              1.70 m
Weight:              60 kg
Peak flow:           510 dm³/min
Resting pulse rate:  75 beats per min
Pulse rate after four minutes exercise:
Time (min) after exercise:   Pulse rate (beats per 30 seconds):
1  62
2  48
3  38

Other observations: Liz wishes that she had time to do more exercise.

Instead of, or as well as, using any of the case studies above, you could prepare a health plan for one of the following:

▶ yourself

▶ a person you know who would be willing to answer questions on their lifestyle and allow you to make simple health measurements (remember issues of confidentiality, for example, will you need to change the name?)

▶ a named character from a TV 'soap'.

Write an account of the lifestyle and include health measurements as for the case studies. (For the TV character you will, of course, not be able to make health measurements, but you may be able to make observations about their health.)

## TO PRODUCE THE HEALTH PLAN

▶ Calculate BMI (page 259) and Fitness Index (see page 257).

▶ Identify any factors that are having a positive effect on physical, social and emotional health.

▶ Identify risks to physical, social and emotional health, highlighting the ones over which the individual may have control.

▶ Prioritise long- and short-term targets for improvement, including timescales.

▶ Explain the physical, social and emotional effects on the person of achieving the targets.

▶ Explain in a way appropriate to your chosen person, how they can change their behaviour to meet the targets.

▶ Identify potential difficulties in achieving the plan, and propose realistic ways in which they may be overcome.

▶ Select health promotional materials, explaining why they were chosen and others were rejected, and analysing the ways in which the chosen materials will support the plan.

# RESOURCES

There are a number of organisations and websites that give useful information on promoting health and disease. Some of those with information relevant to this chapter are listed below.

### Alcohol Concern
This is the UK national agency of alcohol misuse.
Waterbridge House
32–36 Loman Street
London SE1 OEE
Tel. 020 7928 7377 Fax. 020 7928 4644
www.alcoholconcern.org.uk

### Alcoholics Anonymous
You can look for your local branch of the AA in your telephone directory.
www.alcoholics-anonymous.org

### Central Drugs Prevention Unit
Home Office
Room 354
Horseferry House
Dean Ryle Street
London SW1P 2AW.
Tel. 020 7 217 8631
Will provide a wall chart free of charge which illustrates the major drugs of misuse, and drug taking equipment.

### Contraceptive Education Service
Tel. 020 7636 7866
For general advice on contraception, or how to find a clinic.

### Cyberdiet
This site:
* gives the nutrient content of foods
* gives daily nutrient and energy intake recommendations
* allows you to calculate BMI (see page 257)
* sets goals for weight loss
* gives target heart rates during exercise.
www.cyberdiet.com

### DoH (Department of Health)
The Government department for health
www.doh.gov.uk

### Drinkline

National alcohol helpline – gives confidential advice and information about drinking.
Tel. 0345 32 02 02

### Health Development Agency

Trevelyan House
30 Great Peter St.
London SW1P 2HW
Tel. 020 7413 1985/1987
www.hda-online.org.uk
This agency has replaced the **Health Education Authority**. Its aim is to boost the status of public health by advising on good practice and commissioning new research.

### Jeans for Genes

National fundraising campaign for research into inherited diseases. Website gives useful information on genetic diseases.
www.genesforgenes.com

### National Aids Helpline

Tel. 0800 567 123
A free, 24-hour confidential service that won't show up on your phone bill. Can also give advice on other sexually transmitted diseases.

### National Air Quality Information Archive Bulletin System

Gives current hourly pollution levels for each UK region and a 24-hour forecast.
www.aeat.co.uk/netcen/airqual/forecast.html

### National Asthma Campaign

Providence House
Providence Place
London N1 ONT
Tel. 020 7226 2260 Fax. 020 7704 0740
Can provide information on **peak flow** measurements.

### National Asthma Campaign Scotland

21 Coates Crescent
Edinburgh EH4 7AF
Tel. 0131 226 2544 Fax. 0131 226 2401
www.asthma.org.uk

## Asthma Helpline

Tel: 0345 01 02 03

Advice given by a team of specialist asthma nurses.

## National Drugs Helpline

Tel: 0800 77 66 00 – in Welsh on 0800 37 11 41.

This gives free, 24-hour confidential advice about drugs, including how to talk to children about drugs, counselling, or information on anything to do with drugs. It can give information about local services available in your area.

## UK National Screening Committee

www.doh.gov.uk/ncs

Advises the Government on all aspects of screening policy. Their website gives background information on their role and explains how screening programmes work.

## National Society for Clean Air (NSCA)

www.nsca.org.uk

## open.gov.uk

This service provides a first entry point to UK public sector information.

www.ukonline.gov.uk

## WHO (World Health Organisation)

www.who.int/home-page/

# Glossary

**anorexia nervosa**
an eating disorder, characterised by severe weight loss.

**blood pressure**
the pressure at which blood flows through the circulatory system

**body mass index (BMI)**
a simple assessment of body mass.
$$BMI = \frac{body\ mass/kg}{(height/m)^2}$$

**bulimia nervosa**
an eating disorder characterised by episodes of compulsive overeating usually followed by self-induced vomiting.

**chronic condition**
a disease of long duration involving very slow changes. It often starts very gradually.

**disease**
a specific condition of ill health, identified as an actual change on the surface or inside some part of the body.

**DNA (deoxyribonucleic acid)**
the molecule that forms the genetic material.

**emotional health**
concerned with being able to express feelings such as fear, joy, grief, frustration and anger. It also includes the ability to cope with anxiety, stress, and depression.

**health promotion**
the process of enabling people to increase their control over, and to improve, their health.

**hygiene**
concerned with preventing disease-causing organisms entering the body.

**illness**
the subjective state of feeling unwell (i.e. how people feel). (Compare with **Disease** and **Sickness**.)

**intellectual health**
this is concerned with the ability to think clearly and rationally. It is closely linked to emotional and social health.

**mutation**
an unpredictable change in genetic material.

**obesity**
the excessive deposit of fat under the skin.

**peak flow**
a measure of how fast you can blow air out of your lungs.

**physical health**
concerned with the physical functioning of the body. It is the easiest aspect of health to measure.

**screening**
a simple test carried out on a large number of apparently healthy people to separate those who probably have a certain disease from those who do not.

**sickness**
reported illness. Involves being treated by a professional and becoming a medical statistic.

**sphygmomanometer**
equipment used for measuring blood pressure.

**social health**
this is concerned with the ability to relate to others and to form relationships.

**social isolation**
a situation in which a person has low levels of social contact.

**vaccine**
a preparation given to a person to stimulate their white blood cells to produce antibodies.

# ANSWERS

**Diet.** page 207

Energy requirements depend on:

▶ age (size)

▶ sex

▶ activity levels.

Reasons for the elderly neglecting their diet:

▶ low income

▶ poor mobility

▶ poor appetite

▶ apathy and depression (e.g. if living alone)

▶ reluctance to change habits.

(You may think of other equally valid answers.)

## Stimulating work, education and leisure activity, page 217

1. (ii) Ways in which pregnancy could cause poor education could include: time missed from school during and immediately after the pregnancy; cost of childcare means mother's education cut short; combining studying and childcare is exhausting.

2. Employment can benefit a person in a number of ways, other than providing an income. For example, some types of employment that involve physical activity may contribute to fitness; a person may feel intellectually stimulated by their employment; it is likely that employment will provide opportunities for socialising and friendship.

## Vaccination, page 221

2. German measles (rubella) can cause serious defects in an unborn baby.

## Illegal drug use, page 226

▶ Don't panic.

▶ Make sure they've got plenty of fresh air.

▶ Try not to leave them alone in case they vomit and choke.

▶ Dial 999 and ask for an ambulance.

▶ Collect up anything that seems to have been used in the drug taking and give them to a member of the ambulance crew.

Sexual behaviour quiz, page 247

1. d)

2. b)

3. g)

Poverty, page 249

Advantage of minimum wage: prevents exploitation of workers.

Disadvantages of minimum wage: may mean employers can afford to employ fewer workers; may be difficult to enforce.

Housing, pages 250

| Health Problem: | Cause(s) |
|---|---|
| Asthma | Damp |
| Bad back | Carrying pushchair/child upstairs |
| Diarrhoea | Inadequate food storage; poor washing facilities (overcrowded and lack of hot water after 10 pm); possibly lack of hygiene in mobile food van. |
| Depression | Overcrowding causing stress; lack of social contact. |

Weight, page 258–259

2. Palin: overweight.

Action: increase exercise/cut back on fats in diet.

Kate: underweight. Action: a higher energy diet is required.

Peter: okay.

BMI, page 258

1. Guy 29 (overweight)

Heather 24 (ideal weight)

Rachel 25 (ideal weight)

2. Main advantage: quick and easy. No calculations.

Main disadvantage: takes no account of taller people having larger waists.

# Understanding Personal Developments and Relationships

# 4

## CHAPTER CONTENT

This chapter will help you learn about:

▶ the stages and patterns of human growth and development
▶ the different factors that can affect human growth and development
▶ the development of self-concept and personal relationships
▶ major life changes and how people deal with them
▶ the role of relationships in personal development.

Health, social care and early years workers need to know about the different ways that people grow and develop throughout their lives. This chapter will help you to find out about the process of human growth and development and the different factors that can affect an individual's experience.

## HUMAN GROWTH AND DEVELOPMENT

**How do individuals grow and develop during each life stage?**

▶ **Growth** is an increase in size and complexity.
▶ **Development** is the process of gaining new skills.

**Milestones**, or **norms**, show what most children can do at a particular age. However, it is important to remember that, although using norms helps us understand patterns of development, each child will, of course, develop in their own unique way and there will be wide variation between individuals. Keep this in mind when using the development tables below.

Throughout a person's life, growth and development should be considered under the following headings:

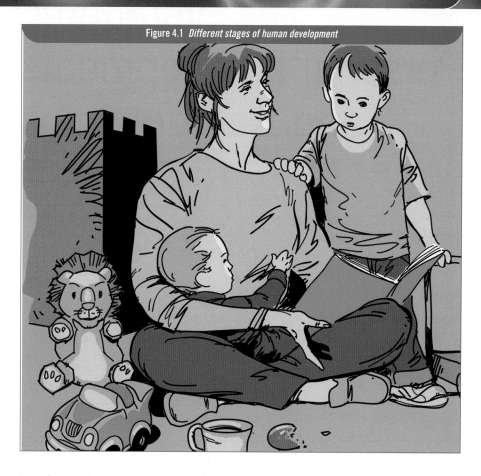

Figure 4.1 *Different stages of human development*

▶ physical

▶ intellectual

▶ emotional

▶ social.

(Remember, the word '**pies**' should help you learn these headings. See page 195–196 in Chapter 3. Each of these types of development are described below.)

Growth and development takes place during each of the five main life stages (Table 4.1).

Table 4.1 *The five main life stages*

| LIFE STAGE | APPROXIMATE AGE RANGE |
|---|---|
| Infancy | 0–3 years |
| Childhood | 4–10 years |
| Puberty and adolescence | 11–18 years |
| Adulthood | 19–65 |
| Old age | 65 and beyond |

# Growth

## Growth in infancy

There are various ways of measuring the growth of a baby (Figure 4.2). The three measurements most commonly made are:

▶ weight

▶ length

▶ head circumference.

A newborn baby, on average:

▶ weighs 3.5 kg

▶ has a length of about 50 cm

▶ has a head circumference of about 35 cm.

Boys are, on average, about 100g heavier than girls, and slightly longer.

---

Figure 4.2  *a) Weighing a baby, b) Measuring the length of a baby, c) Measuring the head circumference of a baby*

**a)**

**b)**

**c)**

The body parts of a baby do not all grow at the same rate. For example, in the first year:

- the **legs** and **arms** grow at a **faster** rate than the rest of the body
- the **head** grows at a **slower** rate than the rest of the body.

Figure 4.3 shows how the differences in growth rates of the various parts of the body leads to changes in the proportions of the body.

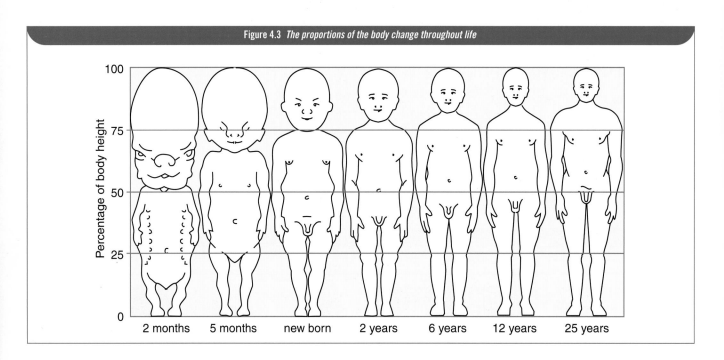

Figure 4.3 *The proportions of the body change throughout life*

# Activity

1. Figure 4.4 shows the average weights, lengths and head circumferences of boy babies.
   (i) Look at this and work out how long it takes for an average baby to double its birth weight. (Give your answer to the nearest month). (Answer on page 335).
   (ii) Many health authorities issue parents with a **Personal Health Record** book to record measurements of their babies. If possible, have a look at one of these books.
2. You may be able to arrange to observe a health visitor weighing babies at a local clinic. (This activity would obviously not be suitable for a whole class, but may be possible for one or two students at a time.)

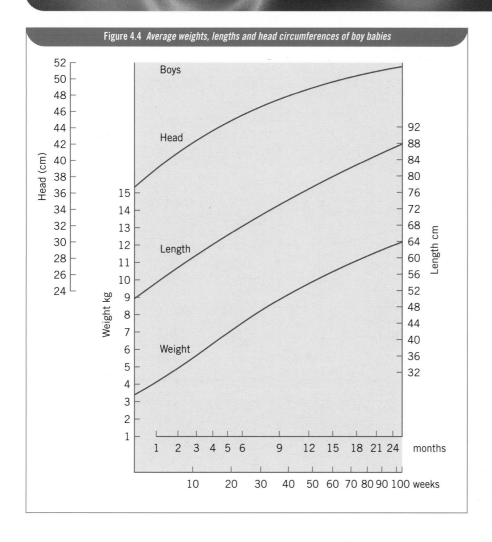

**Figure 4.4** *Average weights, lengths and head circumferences of boy babies*

## Growth in childhood

By the time a child is three years old, their weight is generally about four times their birth weight (Figure 4.4). Figure 4.5 shows growth rate between the ages two and nine. During this time growth takes place at a fairly constant rate, and at a slower rate than the growth between 0–1 years.

The skull and brain have usually reached adult size by the time the child is about five, but after this the child's appearance changes as the upper and lower jaws grow rapidly, and the first set of teeth are replaced by the permanent teeth.

## Growth in puberty and adolescence

In adolescence there is a sudden increase in growth rate and maturity. This produces an adult who would be able to produce and care for young.

Adolescence starts with **puberty**, which is the time during which **secondary sexual characteristics** develop (see Figure 4.6). Puberty

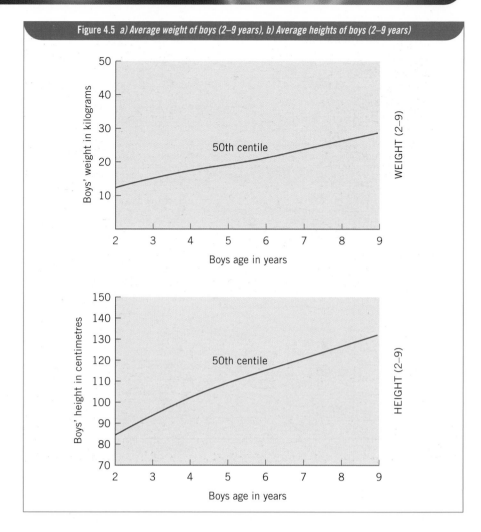

Figure 4.5 a) Average weight of boys (2–9 years), b) Average heights of boys (2–9 years)

usually starts at about 10 in girls, and 12 in boys. By late teens the changes are usually complete.

The increase in growth rate in **adolescence** is known as the **second growth spurt**. This is different in males and females.

▶ In girls the growth spurt usually occurs between about 11 and 12 years, but in boys it is usually between about 13 and 15 years old.

▶ In boys the growth spurt lasts longer than in girls, which means men are generally larger than women.

## Growth in adulthood

By the end of adolescence the body is physically and sexually mature. Although growth no longer takes place, physical changes to the body continue as the body ages.

The **menopause** occurs in women, usually between about 45 and 55. After this they do not produce eggs which means they can no longer become pregnant. Men, however, can produce sperm and thus father children into old age.

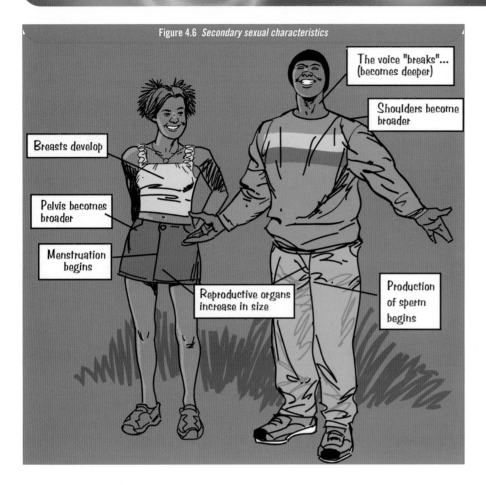

Figure 4.6 *Secondary sexual characteristics*

## Growth in old age

Figure 4.7 shows how the main body systems deteriorate with age. Despite these changes, it is important that elders are encouraged to approach the ageing process with a positive attitude. Improved health care (among other factors) has increased life expectancy and the quality of life in old age, and their wealth of experience allows elderly people to make valuable contributions.

# Physical development

Figure 4.8 shows that the physical skills which develop throughout life can be divided into two main areas: gross motor skills and fine motor skills.

## Physical development in infancy

Table 4.2 shows the development of both gross motor skills and fine manipulative skills in infancy.

## Physical development in childhood

Table 4.3 shows the development of both gross motor skills and fine manipulative skills in childhood.

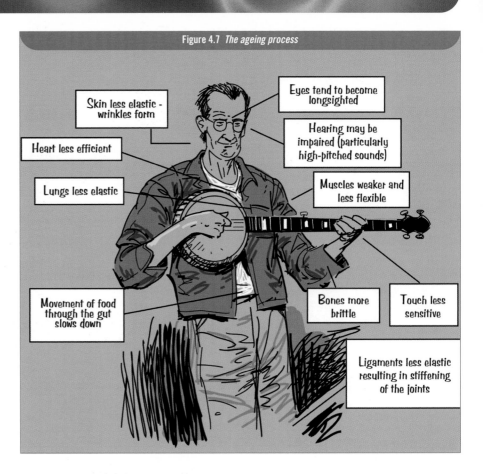

Figure 4.7 *The ageing process*

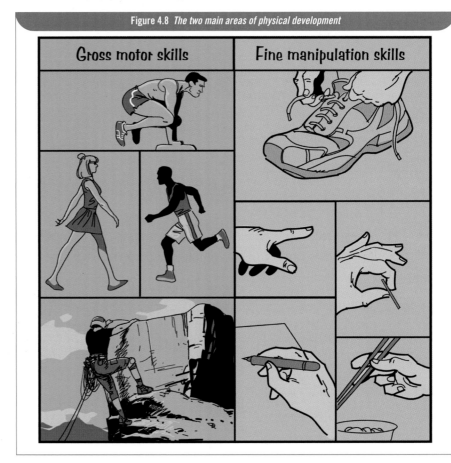

Figure 4.8 *The two main areas of physical development*

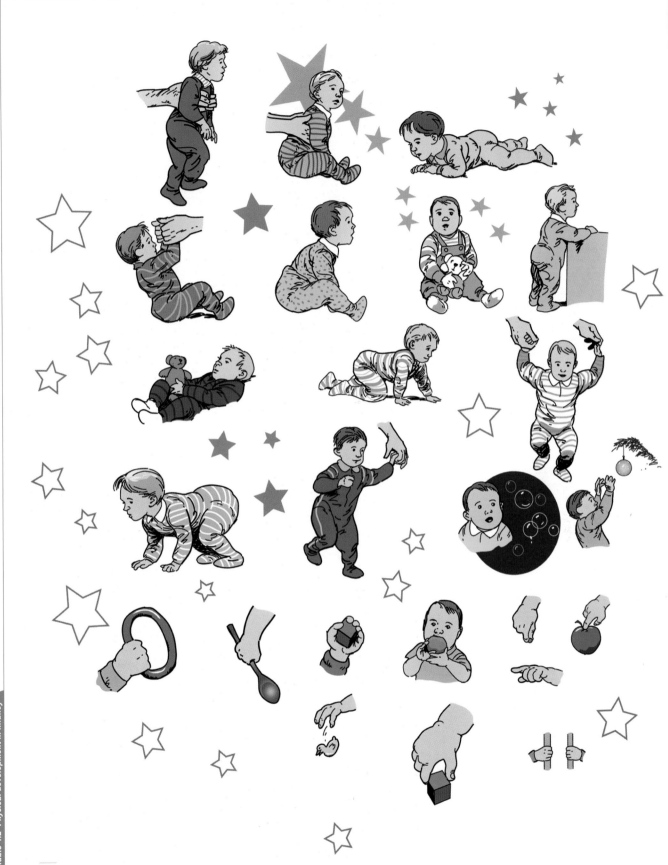

Table 4.2 Physical development in infancy

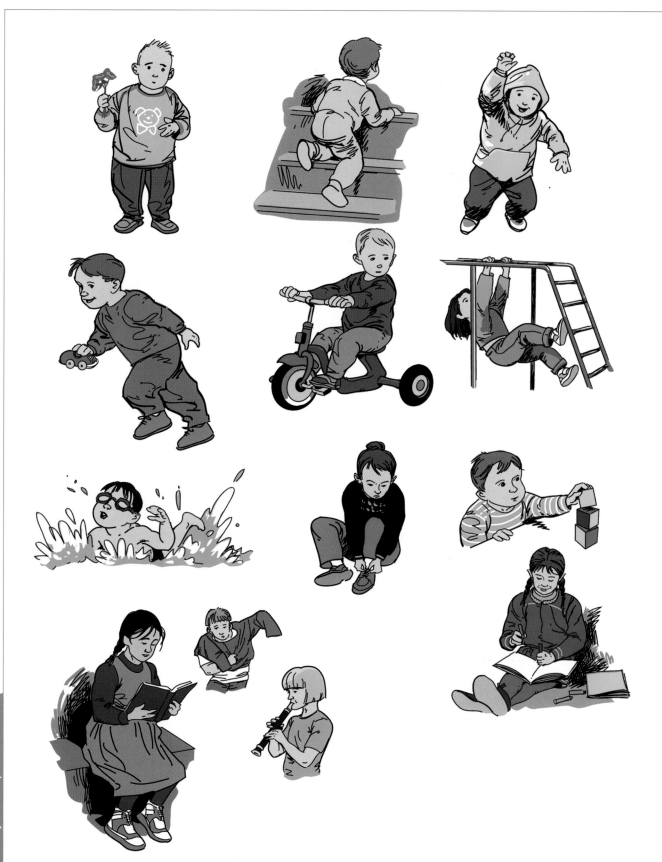

Table 4.3 *Physical development in childhood*

## Physical development in puberty and adolescence, adulthood, old age

By the time the nervous system is fully developed, all the main developmental milestones will have been reached. However, even in later life, people may learn new gross motor skills and fine manipulative skills.

# Activity

1. Read the list below of examples of skills which may be acquired in adulthood. Which are gross motor skills and which are fine manipulative skills?
   ▶ Rollerblading
   ▶ Embroidery
   ▶ Skiing
   ▶ Playing the flute
2. Can you think of any physical skills you have learnt since childhood?

# Intellectual development

Intellectual development refers to the development of the parts of the brain concerned with:

▶ perception (absorbing information about the environment through the senses of sight, hearing, touch, smell and taste)

▶ acquiring knowledge

▶ reasoning

▶ understanding.

Every brain cell a person has is present at their birth. During childhood the brain grows very quickly. By the age of one year, the baby's brain is already three-quarters of its adult size and rapid development continues until middle childhood.

### Intellectual development in infancy

Table 4.4 shows some of the stages of intellectual development in infancy.

### Intellectual development in childhood

Table 4.5 shows some of the stages of intellectual development in childhood.

| Age | Development |
|---|---|
| 0–4 weeks | Babies receive information about the world through their senses.<br>*Touch* Their faces, abdomens, hands and soles of feet are particularly sensitive.<br>*Hearing* Newborn babies turn towards a sound. By 2 weeks old they will stop crying and listen to a human voice.<br><br>*Taste* Like sweet tastes.<br>*Smell* Turn to the smell of the breast.<br>*Sight* Can focus on objects about 200m away, but probably don't see colour.<br>They will initiate facial expressions. |
| 4–16 weeks | Recognise different speech sounds.<br>By 3 months they can imitate low or high pitched sounds. |
| 4–5 months | Can reach objects, showing that they can judge distances.<br>Know the difference between two- and three-dimensional objects. |
| 5–6 months | Recognise familiar objects, e.g. feeding bottle.<br>Can coordinate movements such as reaching or grasping.<br>Develop favourite tastes in food. |
| 6–9 months | Understands signs (e.g. bib means food is coming)<br>Understands that objects are permanant (e.g. when a toy is covered with cloth it still exists.) |
| 9 months–1 year | Memory develops. Can anticipate the future, so can understand daily routines.<br>Can imitate events after they have finished. (e.g. initiate a temper tantrum they saw a friend have the day before.) |

Table 4.4 Intellectual development in infants

| Age | Development |
|---|---|
| 1–4 years | Talking develops.<br>Pretend play develops.<br>Can take part in simple games.<br>Learn to draw and make models.<br>May start to enjoy music.<br>Find it difficult to see things from another's point of view, but this will start to develop. |
| 4–7 years | Language is well established.<br>Reading and writing develop.<br>Concepts of measurement develop (e.g. length, time, weight).<br>An understanding of number develops.<br>Can help younger children play.<br>Start to develop an understanding of 'right' and 'wrong'. |
| 9 years onwards | Develops an understanding of abstract concepts such as justice, good versus evil. |

Table 4.5 Intellectual development in childhood

## Intellectual development in puberty and adolescence into adulthood

The way in which adolescents and adults think may differ in a number of ways from the way children think. For example:

▶ **Thinking about possibilities**: young children rely heavily on their senses to apply reasoning, whereas adolescents are more likely to think about alternative possibilities that are not directly observable.

▶ **Thinking ahead**: adolescence is the time when young people start to plan ahead. Younger children may look forward to a holiday, for example, but are not able to focus on the preparation required.

▶ **Thinking about thought**: adolescents can think about their own thought processes in an increasingly complex way. They are also able to think more about other people's points of view.

▶ **Thinking beyond conventional limits**: issues such as morality, religion and politics, which are probably not considered by children, are more likely thought about by adolescents.

## Intellectual development in old age

In old age there may be changes in memory, but only in certain aspects. Long-established skills, such as money management, playing a musical instrument or gardening, remain unaffected by old age. The memory for names and everyday activities, however may be affected. Sometimes, an old person may find it difficult to distinguish between a real and an imagined event. For example, some elderly people may believe they have turned the gas off, when in reality they have only **thought** about turning it off.

The ability to recall events from the distant past improves slightly into middle age, and by the age of 60 shows only a slight decline.

### Activity

Read through the four examples above of how an adolescent's, or adult's, thinking may differ from a child's thinking. For each, can you remember any examples of occasions on which you have demonstrated this type of thinking?

### Activity

Discuss how Christine should react. Can you think of strategies to help elderly people remember important actions and events?

## CASE STUDY ONE: CHRISTINE

Christine goes to visit her elderly mother who lives very close to her. As she arrives, she finds her mother returning from a day trip. They go into her mother's house together to find that the gas cooker has been left on. A saucepan and its contents have been ruined, but there is no lasting damage.

# Emotional and social development

**Emotional development** involves the development of **self-image** and **identity** (p 312), and the ways in which an individual makes sense of emotions in themselves, and of feelings towards other people.

**Social development** involves the growth of the individual's **relationship** with others and the development of social skills.

## Emotional and social development in infancy

Table 4.6 shows some of the stages in emotional and social development in infancy.

## Emotional and social development in childhood

Table 4.7 shows some of the stages of emotional and social development in childhood.

## Emotional and social development in adolescence and puberty

Adolescence is a period when most young people are working towards their own independence. They want to be able to increas-

Table 4.6 Emotional and social development in infants

| | |
|---|---|
| Birth – 4 weeks | Enjoyment of feeding and cuddling.<br>The baby shows pleasure, e.g. at bathtime, with whole body movements. |
| 4–8 weeks | Responds by smiling at an adult.<br>Recognises face of preferred adult. Turns towards someone speaking. |
| 8–12 weeks | Longer periods of being awake.<br>Fixes eyes on carer's face when feeding. |
| 4–5 months | Sleep patterns have developed.<br>Knows she has only one mother, and shows distress if several images of the mother are shown at one time. |
| 6–9 months | More wary of strangers.<br>Offers toys to others.<br>Shows distress when main carer leaves.<br>Becomes more aware of others' feelings. e.g. will cry if brother cries: will laugh if others laugh. |
| 9–12 months | Likes to be near familiar adult.<br>Will play alone for long periods.<br>Shows definite likes and dislikes, e.g. at mealtime or bedtime.<br>Imitates other people, e.g. clapping or waving. |

| | |
|---|---|
| 1–2 years | Starts to learn what hurts and upsets their family, and what brings pleased responses.<br>A longer memory develops.<br>Express needs in words and gestures. |
| 2–3 years | Develops ability to say how s/he is feeling.<br>Pretend play helps a child develop a sense of what other people are feeling. |
| 3–4 years | Becomes aware of being male or female.<br>Makes friends.<br>Learns to negotiate with others. |
| 4–8 year | Can hide feelings.<br>Can think about the feelings of others.<br>Can take responsibility (e.g. will help younger children). |

*Table 4.7 Emotional and social development in childhood*

ingly make their own decisions, test the limits of authority and express their own individuality. It is also a time when peer pressure is at its highest. During the early part of adolescence, young people are likely to be more self-conscious and more self-critical than before.

## Emotional and social development in adulthood

Adulthood has been described as a state of **maturity**. A mature individual is considered to have the following attributes:

▶ stable emotional behaviour

▶ an accurate self-concept (see page 312)

▶ satisfying relationships

▶ a realistic estimation of future goals.

These attributes will help when it comes to dealing with the inevitable life changes which will be faced in adulthood (see page 320).

## Emotional and social development in old age

Three different theories of ageing help to explain some of the emotional and social changes in this period of life.

1. **Erikson's psycho-social theory** suggests that there are two conflicting points of view in old age. These are illustrated in Figure 4.15. Successful ageing depends on the individual adopting the more positive view of ageing.

2. The **social disengagement theory** (Figure 4.16) suggests that the following social changes take place in old age:

## Activity

**Discussion point:**
It is said that attractiveness and peer acceptance are more important in the development of self-esteem during adolescence than other attributes, such as being good at sports or good at academic subjects. Do you agree with this?

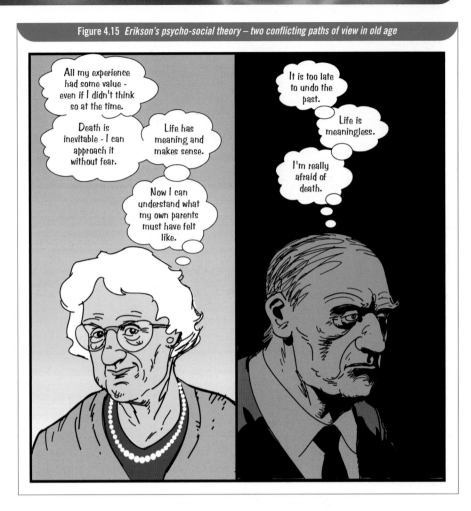

Figure 4.15 *Erikson's psycho-social theory – two conflicting paths of view in old age*

- **Society withdraws from the individual**, for example:
  - there is compulsory retirement, usually at the age of 65
  - children grow up, leave home and have families of their own
  - friends, or maybe the spouse, die.
- **The individual withdraws from society**, for example:
  - there is a reduction in social contacts and activity
  - life becomes more solitary.

It is suggested that the decrease in social and emotional responsibilities in the later years leads to contentment and so these changes are beneficial. Others, however, believe that the changes are harmful and are caused by the negative attitude in society towards elderly people.

3. The **activity theory** (Figure 4.17) proposes that successful ageing involves staying active and participating in as many social activities as possible.

Figure 4.16 *Social disengagement theory*

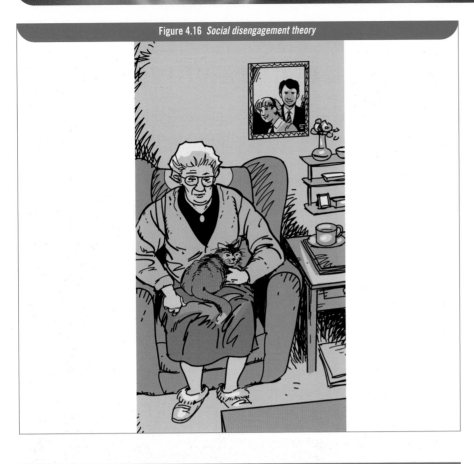

Figure 4.17 *Activity theory*

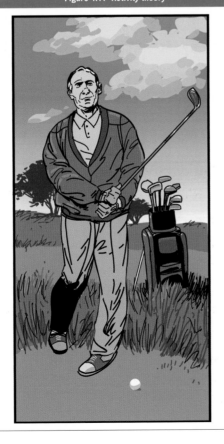

## Activity

Look at Figures 4.16 and 4.17 which illustrate the social disengagement theory and activity theory respectively. Think of specific elderly people and decide which theory you think describes them most accurately.

# FACTORS THAT AFFECT GROWTH AND DEVELOPMENT

What factors affect human growth and development and how can they influence an individual's health, well-being and opportunities?

As explained in Chapter 3, there are a number of factors that contribute both positively (pages 201–223) and negatively (pages 223–252) to health and well-being. These factors can cause individual differences in patterns of growth and development. The factors may be:

▶ physical

▶ social and emotional

▶ economic

▶ environmental.

There is a summary of these factors in Figure 4.18.

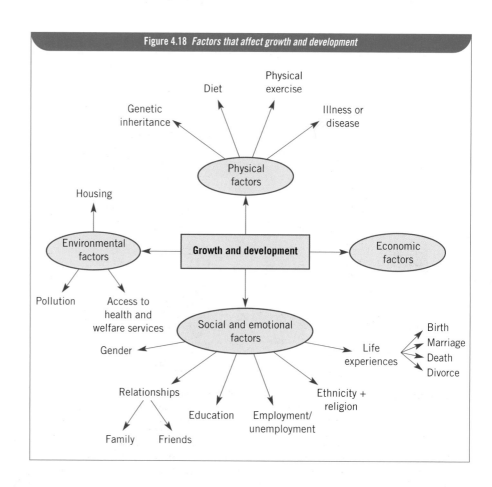

**Figure 4.18 Factors that affect growth and development**

The different factors may interrelate and can affect a person's:

▶ self-esteem (see page 321)
▶ physical and mental health
▶ employment prospects
▶ level of education.

# Physical factors

## Genetic inheritance

(See also pages 223–225, on *Genetically inherited diseases and conditions.*)

The genes an individual inherits from their parents will obviously affect their growth and development. Figure 4.19 shows how a person's height can be predicted from the heights of the parents.

## Diet

The sections on *A balanced diet* (pages 202–207) and *An unbalanced, poor quality or inadequate diet* (page 236) explain the influence of nutrition on health and well-being. Average heights in the UK

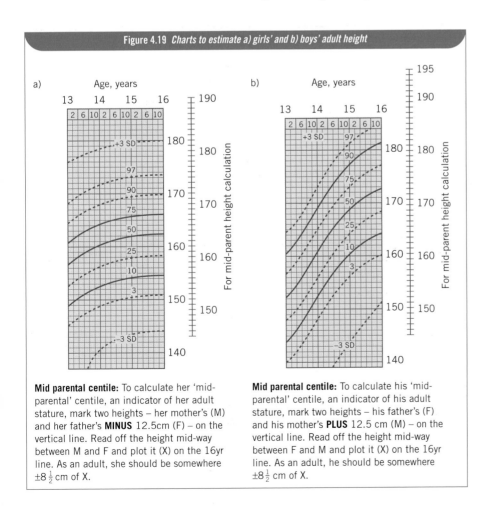

**Figure 4.19** *Charts to estimate a) girls' and b) boys' adult height*

**Mid parental centile:** To calculate her 'mid-parental' centile, an indicator of her adult stature, mark two heights – her mother's (M) and her father's **MINUS** 12.5cm (F) – on the vertical line. Read off the height mid-way between M and F and plot it (X) on the 16yr line. As an adult, she should be somewhere ±8½ cm of X.

**Mid parental centile:** To calculate his 'mid-parental' centile, an indicator of his adult stature, mark two heights – his father's (F) and his mother's **PLUS** 12.5 cm (M) – on the vertical line. Read off the height mid-way between F and M and plot it (X) on the 16yr line. As an adult, he should be somewhere ±8½ cm of X.

increased in the last century, for example, in 1750 the average young male height was about 160 cm, and in 1980 it was 176 cm. It is thought that improved diet is the main reason for this increase in height. Poor nutrition is common in areas of poverty, and it can be seen that in poorer countries the average adult height is less than that in richer countries.

### Physical activity

The sections on *Regular exercise* (pages 212–213) and *Lack of regular physical exercise* (page 244) explain the influence of physical activity on health and well-being.

Exercise is essential for children's growth and development for a number of reasons:

▶ it strengthens muscles, bones and joints

▶ it improves balance, co-ordination, flexibility and posture

▶ it reduces the chance of heart disease in later life

▶ it develops a child's self-esteem by creating a strong sense of purpose and self-fulfilment

▶ team sports teach a child how to interact and cooperate with others.

### Experience of illness or disease

Serious illness or disease can affect all aspects of growth and development. As well as having physical effects, poor health can limit a young person's education, or an older person's employment prospects.

(See also *Genetically inherited diseases and conditions* in Chapter 3 on pages 223–225).

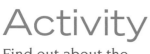

**Activity**

Find out about the provision of education for children in hospital.

## Social and emotional factors

The ways in which individuals grow and develop are not only influenced by biological and physical factors, but are affected, within society, by the kind of 'training' for social life (**socialisation**) people receive through their relationships with others. **Social factors** that affect personal development describe the patterns in, and expectations of, social behaviour which may affect, for instance, people's health, their employment prospects, their level of education and their self-esteem. The groups people are part of (families, friends, ethnic, religious or cultural groups, sex and age categories, such as young boys or adult women, community, work or school-based groups) will have significant impact on their lives.

## Gender

(See the section on *Gender* on page 315, below)

There are a number of health differences between males and females, for example:

▸ women live five years longer, on average, than men

▸ more women than men are either underweight or obese

▸ girls and women are more likely than boys and men to experience depression and to have eating disorders.

There is debate over the causes of these differences. It is difficult to determine the relative importance of genetic and biological factors compared with social and economic factors.

> ## Activity
>
> In recent years, girls have outperformed boys in national exams. Discuss the possible reasons for this.

## Family relationships and friendships

The section below on *The effects of relationships on personal development* (pages 300–311) explains how relationships play a key part in an individual's social and emotional development during each life stage.

## Educational experiences

The section in Chapter 3 on *Stimulating work, education and leisure activity* (pages 216–217) explains the importance of education in health and well-being. The section on *Education* (page 317) explains how it affects an individual's self-concept.

A poor education is likely to affect a person's life opportunities. In 2000, figures supplied by the major examining boards in this country showed that 2.1% of young people sitting GCSEs received no award whatsoever. Young people from poorer areas of the country are much more likely to leave school with fewer qualifications and much less likely to go onto higher education. Those people are likely to suffer greater job insecurity, poorer working conditions and to suffer more unemployment and receive a lower income. Although there are exceptions, for most people their schooling affects their future economic status and income.

## Employment/unemployment

The sections in Chapter 3 on *Stimulating work, education and leisure activity* (pages 216–217) and *Unemployment* explain the importance of employment in health, well-being and life opportunities.

## Ethnicity and religion

Ethnicity is the shared identity which arises from a common culture, religion or tradition. An independent inquiry into inequalities in health, published in 1998, confirmed that there were many indications of poorer health among the minority ethnic groups in England.

There are many ways in which ethnicity and religion may influence health, self-esteem and life opportunities, such as education and employment. For example, there are different cultural traditions about:

▶ diet

▶ religious practices (such as circumcision)

▶ preferences for types of medical treatment

▶ birth and death customs

▶ sexual attitudes and roles

▶ washing and personal hygiene routines.

**Discrimination** is the unfair treatment of a person, or group, because of a negative view of some, or all, of their characteristics. Racial discrimination is well researched, and unfortunately all too common in Britain today. The effects of discrimination can be both long-term, resulting in patterns of disadvantage for whole groups in the population, or short-term, resulting in immediate feelings of anger and/or loss of self-esteem or self-confidence. (See also *Ways of obtaining care services* on page 112).

### Life experiences

The section on *The effects of life events on personal development* (pages 320–334) explains how experiences such as marriage, divorce, the birth of a sibling or child, or the death of a friend or relative, can affect an individual's development.

## Economic factors

Economic factors affect personal development because people need resources (money, income, wealth) to pay for things that are essential, such as food, clothing and housing. People may also want further resources for items that they desire but are not essential, such as designer-label clothing, meals in restaurants or expensive holidays. The ways in which people are able to obtain and use their money will have a significant effect on their health, welfare and self-esteem. The sections in Chapter 3 on *Adequate financial resources* (page 216) and *Poverty* (page 248) explain the importance of economic factors in health, well-being and life opportunities.

# Activity

Game – wants or needs?

### Step One

Look at Table 4.8. You will see that there are a number of suggestions for the **economic resources** we may **want** or **need** to live healthily and happily in this society.

### Step Two

Make a photocopy of Table 4.8 for each small group playing the game, and cut out the 28 suggestion boxes. Each group should then, after discussion, place each suggestion into one of two piles labelled as follows:

1. Economic resources we **need** to live healthily and happily.
2. Economic resources we may **want** to live healthily and happily.

**No suggestion should be placed in either category unless all group members agree.**
Where there is a difference in opinion, the members of the group must justify their choice and attempt to persuade the others that their choice is the right one. If no agreement can be reached, the reasons should be recorded by the group and that suggestion omitted from the final piles.

### Step Three

Each group tells the others which suggestions they have placed in their lists and differences can be noted and discussed. The whole class can decide on where any omitted suggestions from each group should go.

### Step Four

Follow up this game by researching the following questions.

1. What is the average annual income, before tax, of:
   ▶ a single employed man in his twenties in the UK?
   ▶ a single employed woman in his twenties in the UK?
   ▶ a married man in employment?
   ▶ a married woman in employment?
   For each of the categories above, work out how much the **annual** income works out at **per week**.
2. What income from **social security** could an unemployed man or woman in their twenties expect to receive per week in the UK today?
3. What does the current state pension pay, per week to:
   ▶ a single man or woman?
   ▶ a married couple?

| A | B | C | D |
|---|---|---|---|
| **1** Enough income to buy (and replace when worn out/outgrown) a set of basic clothing from second-hand/charity shops or similar, e.g. jumble sales: Approx. **£200.00** per person per year. | **1** Enough income to make (sew, knit etc.) most of your own clothes and to buy the rest. Approx. **£300.00** per person per year. | **1** Enough income to buy (and replace when worn out/outgrown) a set of new basic clothing from high street stores or equivalent, e.g. mail order. Approx. **£600.00** per person per year. | **1** Enough income to buy (and replace when worn out/outgrown) a set of clothing from designer shops/with designer lables. Approx **£1200.00** per person per year. |
| **2** Enough income to afford a weekly food/household goods bills of **£20.00–£30.00** per person. | **2** Enough income to afford a weekly food/household goods bill of **£30.00–£40.00** per person. | **2** Enough income to afford a weekly food/household goods bill of **£40.00–£50.00** per person. | **2** Enough income to afford to spend as much as you like on food and household goods plus resturant and take-away bills. |
| **3** Enough income to afford to buy, after all other essentials have been paid for, up to 4 second-class postage stamps a week. Approx. **£1.00–£2.00** per person. | **3** Enough income to afford to buy, after all other essentials have been paid for, birthday/Christmas/other religious festival presents for close family. Approx. **£80.00** per person per year. | **3** Enough income to afford to buy, after all other essentials have been paid for, up to ten units of alcohol a week and/or twenty cigarettes a day. Approx. **£35.00–50.00** per person per week. | **3** Enough income to afford to buy personal private health insurance. Between **£500.00–1000.00** per person per year. |
| **4** Enough income to buy, insure and maintain a second hand pedal bicycle with safety helmet and puncture kit. Approx. **£150.00** per person in the year the bicycle is bought. | **4** Enough annual income to afford to pay off a monthly loan on, tax, insure, service and buy petrol for a small second-hand car. Approx. **£1800.00** per person in the year the car is bought. | **4** Enough annual income to afford to pay off a monthly loan on, tax, insure, service and buy petrol for a small new car. Approx. **£4000.00** per person in the year the car is bought. | **4** Enough income to afford to buy outright, tax, insure, service and run a new car. Anything above **£12,000.00** in the year the car is bought. |
| **5** Enough income to rent a room in a hostel or night shelter. | **5** Enough income to rent a flat/house from a council, a housing association, private landlord or a co-operative. | **5** Enough income to borrow money from a building society, bank or other lender (this is called a mortgage) to buy a house or flat. You will usually be allowed to borrow two and a half to three times your annual gross income, i.e. before tax. | **5** Enough income to buy your house outright. |
| **6** Enough income to afford a weekly T.V. rental payment and annual T.V. license bill. Approx. **£200.00** a year per person. | **6** Enough income to afford to buy a new T.V. and video and pay the annual T.V. license fee. Approx. **£300.00–400.00** per person in the year the T.V. and video were bought. | **6** Enough income to buy a home computer and software and pay for fax, e-mail and Internet services plus subscriptions to satellites, cable and digital T.V. Approx. **£1500.00–2000.00** in the year the computer was bought. | **6** Enough income to afford to buy outright any combination of T.V., video, computer, fax games console, software, printers etc. the individual or family desires. Approx. **£5000.00+** in the year the items are bought. |
| **7** Employment pay and/or social security benefit/pension which gives an income (after tax) of **£80.00** plus housing benefit per person per week. | **7** Employment pay and/or social security benefit/pension which gives an income (after tax) of **£130.00–250.00** a week. | **7** Employment pay and/or social security benefit/pension which gives an income (after tax) of **£400.00–500.00** per person per week. | **7** Income and earnings which give a weekly income (after tax) of more than **£600.00** per person per week. |

Table 4.8 Suggestion boxes – wants or needs?

## Income, wealth and poverty

The game above shows that there is no easy way to work out how much money, income or wealth is needed for a healthy and happy life.

Many people's main **income** is wages from employment, but other sources of income include benefits, pensions, interest from savings and dividends from shares.

**Wealth** means something slightly different from income because it refers to the total value of the possessions held by an individual (or society). Some possessions, such as a small business, factory or farm, can be a source of income for the people they belong to.

Just as it is difficult to work out the differences between **wants** and **needs**, so it is difficult to define and measure **poverty**. Poverty is a state in which, for an individual or family, there is either a lack of resources sufficient to maintain a healthy existence (absolute poverty) or a lack of resources sufficient to achieve a standard of living considered acceptable in that particular society (relative poverty).

# Environmental factors

### Housing conditions

The section in Chapter 3 on *Inadequate housing* (pages 241–250) explains the importance of housing in health and well-being.

### Pollution

The section in Chapter 3 on *Environmental pollution* (pages 251–252) explains the detrimental effect that pollution can have on health and well-being.

### Access to health and welfare services

In the UK, the National Health Service was set up to provide health for all. However, people do not have equal access to health and welfare services. Some of the social and economic factors already discussed can make a difference to the type of treatment or service people receive. This may then affect their health, employment prospects and view of themselves. For instance:

▶ People with physical disabilities, the elderly or people with young children may find it difficult to manage the journey to hospitals or clinics. If they are also living in poverty, they may be unable to pay transport costs and to arrange the necessary child care to allow them to visit a doctor or attend a clinic. While 11% of the population pays for private health insurance, which gives them access to private health treatment, others have to wait up to four days for an appointment with their GP, or months for a hospital operation.

▶ NHS rules mean that it is difficult for the homeless to register with a GP because they do not have a postal address, although some doctors do register homeless people by giving the surgery address on the form required. The fact that the homeless are up to 25 times more likely to die early than the average citizen, supports the view that it is the most vulnerable groups that have the least access to health care.

▶ In rural areas, poor public transport may put some people off visiting health professionals.

▶ Certain ethnic groups are less likely to use health services and, even when they do, they may find that language difficulties prevent them from obtaining the most effective health care.

▶ Men appear less willing to use preventative health care than women.

▶ The elderly are sometimes discriminated against in access to health care and health treatments.

▶ The availability of health care varies throughout the country. For example, waiting times for hospital treatment; the drugs prescribed; the availability of expertise and the provision of specialist treatment centres for conditions such as cancer, differs from one area to another.

# THE EFFECTS OF RELATIONSHIPS ON PERSONAL DEVELOPMENT

Throughout our lives, from birth until death, we are in relationships and these take many forms.

Key relationships that occur during our lives include the following:

▶ family relationships – with parents, siblings, and other family members

▶ friendships

▶ intimate personal and sexual relationships

▶ working relationships.

## Family relationships

The experience of living as part of a family is something that most people have at some time in their life. The family can be defined as 'a social group linked by ties of blood and marriage', but nowadays family forms vary considerably. The nuclear family consists of one man, one woman and their dependent children.

We can see that the number of single parents has increased and the numbers of people living on their own has also increased.

The family has been traditionally seen as providing the following functions:

**Activity**

Table 4.9 shows the type of households and family forms in Great Britain between 1961 and 2000. Look at the table and identify the changes you see.

| Great Britain | 1961 | 1971 | 1981 | Percentages 1991 | 2000[1] |
|---|---|---|---|---|---|
| **One person** | | | | | |
| Under state pension age | 4 | 6 | 8 | 11 | 14 |
| Over state pension age | 7 | 12 | 14 | 16 | 15 |
| **Two or more unrelated adults** | 5 | 4 | 5 | 3 | 3 |
| **One family households** | | | | | |
| Couple[2] | | | | | |
| No children | 26 | 27 | 26 | 28 | 29 |
| 1–2 dependent children[3] | 30 | 26 | 25 | 20 | 19 |
| 3 or more dependent children[3] | 8 | 9 | 6 | 5 | 4 |
| Non-dependent children only | 10 | 8 | 8 | 8 | 6 |
| Lone parent[2] | | | | | |
| Dependent children[3] | 2 | 3 | 5 | 6 | 6 |
| Non-dependent children only | 4 | 4 | 4 | 4 | 3 |
| **Multi-family households** | 3 | 1 | 1 | 1 | 1 |
| **All households[4]** | | | | | |
| (= 100%)(millions) | 16.3 | 18.6 | 20.2 | 22.4 | 23.9 |

1 At Spring 2000.
2 Other individuals who were not family members may also be included.
3 May also include non-dependent children.
4 Includes couples of the same gender in 2000, but percentages are based on totals excluding this group.

*Source*: Labour Force Survey, Office for National Statistics

**Table 4.9** *Types of household and family forms in Great Britain, 1961–2000*

# Activity

Table 4.10 shows the percentage of children living in different family types. Describe the patterns that you see.

▶ teaching children values, attitudes and rules of social behaviour

▶ supporting the emotional development of the child from infancy to adulthood

▶ offering stability and security (this could include economic support)

▶ protecting the health and well-being of all its members.

Family relationships are said to be **primary relationships** because the people in the family know each other very well, they relate to each other on an informal basis, and one person in the relationship cannot be replaced.

Family relationships are affected by death, divorce and the separation of parents. Since 1990–91 there has been an increase in cohabitation among all age groups. Men are more likely than women to be single, but less likely to be divorced, separated or widowed. This reflects the evidence that men are more likely than women to remarry after losing a partner through death or divorce, and women are more likely to outlive their husbands.

We can see from this table that the traditional couple family is still the most common type of family in which dependent children live.

| Great Britain | 1972 | 1981 | 1991–92 | Percentages 2000[1] |
|---|---|---|---|---|
| **Couple families** | | | | |
| 1 child | 16 | 18 | 17 | 17 |
| 2 children | 35 | 41 | 37 | 38 |
| 3 or more children | 41 | 29 | 28 | 26 |
| **Lone mother families** | | | | |
| 1 child | 2 | 3 | 5 | 6 |
| 2 childen | 2 | 4 | 7 | 7 |
| 3 or more children | 2 | 3 | 6 | 6 |
| **Lone father families** | | | | |
| 1 child | – | 1 | – | 1 |
| 2 or more children | 1 | 1 | 1 | 1 |
| **All dependent children[2]** | 100 | 100 | 100 | 100 |

1 At Spring 2000.
2 In Spring 2000, includes cases where the dependent child is a family unit, for example, a foster child.
   *Source*: General Household Survey and Labour Force Survey, Office for National Statistics

Table 4.10 The percentage of dependent children living in different family types, 1972–2000

## Geneograms

**Geneograms** are a type of diagram used to show the structure of a family and the relationships between the different members. They show family trees in diagram form. The symbols that are used in geneograms are shown in Figure 4.20.

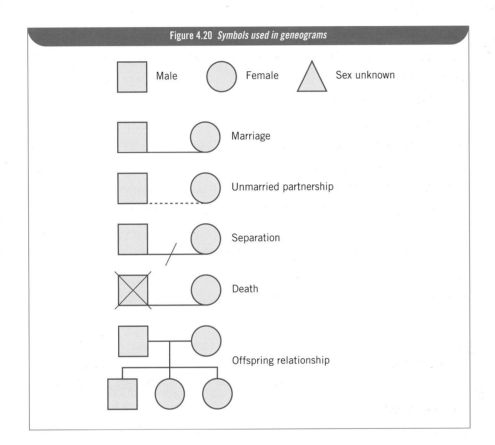

**Figure 4.20** *Symbols used in geneograms*

# Activity

### Draw a geneogram of the following family

David (55) is cohabiting with Jean (55). Jean's husband John, died, but David is divorced from his wife. Jean has three children, one of whom is Phil (35), who is married to Clare (30). They have a son, Thomas, who is two years old. Jean's daughter Louise (32) is single and lives on her own. Jean's second son Paul (30) lives with his partner Judy. David has one son, Robert (18) who lives with his mother Sue (50) and her live-in partner Simon. David's mother Beatrice (90) is still alive and lives on her own. She is a widow.

We can see from this example that family relationships can be quite complicated, especially when members have separated or made new relationships.

Look at the activity again and think about possible areas where there can be negative and positive effects of living in such a family.

## Discussion

Children from a marriage may find it difficult to cope when their parents divorce and find new partners. Women, such as Jean, who have brought up a family, may find it difficult to build a relationship with their partner's children, especially if they are younger. Jean may also feel responsible for supporting Beatrice. The children of widowed parents are often very protective and can be suspicious of a new partner.

Figure 4.21 shows the ages of children of couples who have divorced. We can see from this that many children are involved. Step families account for about 6% of all families with dependent children. There is a tendency for children to remain with their mother after a partnership breaks up. Figure 4.22 shows the composition of step families with dependent children .

Relationships between parents, children, and siblings can have positive effects, but they can also have negative effects.

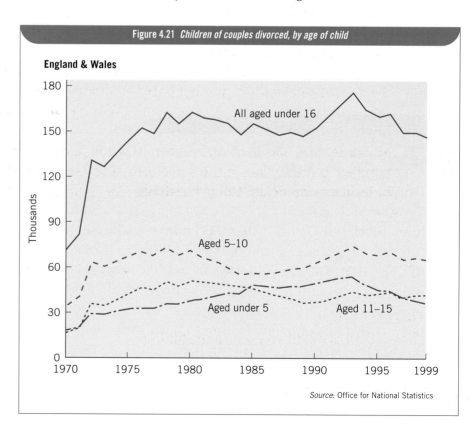

**Figure 4.21 *Children of couples divorced, by age of child***

England & Wales

All aged under 16

Aged 5–10

Aged under 5

Aged 11–15

*Source*: Office for National Statistics

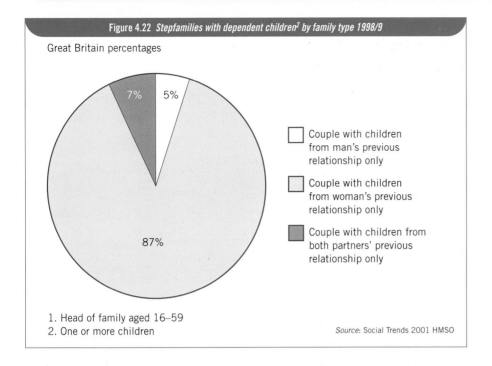

**Figure 4.22** *Stepfamilies with dependent children[2] by family type 1998/9*

Great Britain percentages

7%  5%

87%

- Couple with children from man's previous relationship only
- Couple with children from woman's previous relationship only
- Couple with children from both partners' previous relationship only

1. Head of family aged 16–59
2. One or more children

*Source*: Social Trends 2001 HMSO

# Activity

Identify the negative and positive effects from the following examples.

1. Surinder (8) lives with her parents and grandparents in West London in a small flat above the family business.
2. Merya (14) lives with her mother and older brother. Each weekend she goes to stay with her father and his girlfriend.
3. James (6) is the youngest of four brothers, who are 8, 10, and 12.
4. Susan (30) has just had her first baby. Her mother and mother-in-law are delighted at this event and as they both live nearby they can't wait to give Sue the benefit of their advice.
5. Margaret is 75 and lives on her own. Her son and daughter are married with their own families, but they live in the same area. They see their mother once a week and can help in emergencies. Margaret wishes she could see more of her grandchildren.

We can see from these examples that family relationships are formed

- ▶ between parents
- ▶ between parents or step parents and children
- ▶ between children
- ▶ between other relatives.

# Friendships

Friendships are important social relationships that we choose to establish with other people because we share interests or because we like each other. There is an emotional connection between friends, although it may not be as deep as in families. However, we all know the saying 'you can choose your friends but you cannot choose your family', and not everybody has a close relationship with their family.

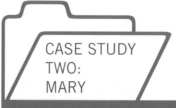

CASE STUDY TWO: MARY

Mary (55) is blind. She was premature (born early) and as a result was blind. When she was 18 months old she was sent to a residential home for blind children. When she was 11 she went to another residential Blind School. Mary says that her mother was very sad that her daughter had to live away from home and she was only home for the holidays. Mary trained as a typist and she is now living in a flat on her own. She still keeps in touch with friends she made when she was at the Blind School. Mary has never married. She has friends who have married and have children. She says her friends are very important to her, as she has known them most of her life. Some of her friends are blind but others are sighted.

## Activity

1. Make a list of your childhood friends (at primary school or in your local area). How many of these do you still see?
2. Which of your current friends do you think you will still be friendly with in 10 years time? Why do you think these friendships will last?

Friends can have close personal relationships, where they can talk about problems and receive emotional support, but we can also have more superficial relationships with people we would not identify as friends. Examples of this type of relationship could be neighbours, members of a church or social group, people we see regularly and may chat to. In this type of relationship you would not discuss personal matters.

As we have seen with Mary's story, close friendships can last a long time. Even if we change schools, move house, change jobs or get married, we will still keep some of our friends.

# Intimate personal and sexual relationships

In early adulthood most people become interested in developing intimate relationships that may lead to stable partnerships and children. Many magazines, books and newspaper articles give advice on how to develop relationships. We have all seen letters in problem pages of magazines and television programmes on relationship difficulties. Close personal relationships can offer emotional support as well as being a way of expressing our feelings sexually.

# Working relationships

Work relationships are usually with people who are not members of our biological family and whose connection with us is more short-term. Work relationships are said to be secondary relationships for the following reasons:

▶ interaction between people is limited to work situations

▶ there are clear rules about how the relationship should be conducted

▶ there are clearly defined social roles (e.g. employer/worker, teacher/student).

Relationships at work can be formal or informal. Formal relationships are those that are based on the work situation, and usually there is a power relationship (between the boss and employee, or the teacher and student). However, fellow workers may have informal relationships, which may be very important if the job is stressful or boring.

Look at Case Study 3. We can see in the example below that Louise has different relationships with colleagues, customers and her boss.

Do you have a part-time job? What type of relationships do you have at work and do they affect how you feel about yourself? If we are being constantly put down by the boss or ignored by fellow workers, this can have a negative effect on how we feel about the job and also how we feel about ourselves. We all need to feel valued and appreciated, and it is important that employers show recognition of our efforts.

**Social role** – the part played by an individual that involves expectations from others, and obligations towards others

## CASE STUDY THREE: LOUISE

Louise (16) is a student at a local college, but she works one evening and all day Saturday at a local supermarket on the till. Several other part-timers are also students, and they chat when they have their coffee break. At Christmas they went out for a meal at a local pub. Louise finds the work boring but she needs the money. She says that the best thing about the job is the people that she works with. Her boss, Neil, told her off last week for being rude to a customer. Some customers are regulars who come to her till and have a chat. Louise enjoys this as it breaks the routine, but Neil told her she cannot do this too much if they are busy, as customers start complaining.

Most jobs have job descriptions that form the basis of the formal contract between the worker and employer. These state the duties of the job. We have seen examples of these in Chapter 2. However, jobs that are based on formal relationships alone would become very unfulfilling for the worker.

Members of professional groups, such as teachers and doctors, have clearly defined standards of behaviour towards their students or patients, and these are formal guidelines that need to be followed. If not, the professional may be disciplined and lose their job. Examples of this would be teachers who use their powerful position to have unlawful sexual relationships with their pupils, or doctors who have sexual relationships with their patients.

We have seen in this section that relationships are an important aspect of our lives. They offer practical and emotional support, and make us feel happy about ourselves.

Relationships change as we get older and our lives change. Change and development can be positive, but it can also be difficult to cope with if we do not have support. If relationships break down, people can feel sad, lonely, angry and negative about themselves. This can lead to behaviour such as drinking too much, smoking and using drugs, over or under eating. People can feel isolated and withdraw from social contact with others. If you feel isolated and upset, this can have an effect on your ability to concentrate on your work or study. People may become depressed and develop physical symptoms such as headaches, tiredness and difficulty in sleeping.

It would seem that supportive relationships with family and friends are very important for our general well-being, and that when these breakdown the effects can be very negative. However, some relationships can have a very negative effect on our personal development.

# Abuse and neglect

Taking care of young children is a very demanding task for all parents. Social workers are sometimes involved when infants fail to thrive. In their role they have to explore the social and emotional support the child is receiving from its parents or parent. The *Children Act* (1989) describes parents' ability to raise their child:

---

*'All parents should provide safety, shelter, space (space to play, and space for privacy for older children), food, income, physical care and health care. Parents should also provide love, security, attention, new experiences, acceptance, education, praise and recognition in order to meet their children's needs.'*

---

Child abuse is one of the most common causes of death in young children in Britain. The *Children Act* was brought in to protect children, but child abuse is still taking place (see Chapter 2). Once social workers identify a child that is at risk from abuse, the child will be put on an **at risk** register, and a close working relationship will be established between the family and the social worker in order to support the parents in their parenting role. This programme could include using a local nursery for the child, bringing in volunteers to support the family (such as the charity Homestart) and parents may be encouraged to go to parenting classes (see Case Study 4).

Children who have been abused have difficulty developing physical and intellectual skills and they may also have problems making relationships in later life.

Abuse and neglect may occur at other times apart from childhood.

**Domestic violence** is seen as a key issue. Men from all social and cultural groups can use violence against women they know. Current research shows that at least one woman in four will experience domestic violence in her lifetime, and one in ten in any one year. Women are more likely to be at risk from an ex-partner.

Women find it difficult to tell someone about the abuse because they feel they may not be believed or they may be blamed in some way.

CASE STUDY THREE: DANIELLE

Danielle has been a volunteer with Homestart for five years. This is her story.

'I have supported a number of families for different periods of time, depending on their needs. One parent had been in care herself and had never had a parent figure from whom to learn parenting skills. One mother had trouble bonding with her baby, another one was struggling with twins, and as I have twins myself I could suggest practical ways to cope. Some mothers had post-natal depression. With all the families I have supported, I feel that the common thread has been the low self-esteem of the mother.'

Volunteers who work for Homestart are all parents themselves and, after a preparation course, they support parents with at least one child under five who are finding it hard to cope.

The effects of an abusive relationship on a woman's personal development can include:

▶ lack of self-esteem

▶ shame and responsibility for the events

▶ loneliness, isolation and an inability to make decisions.

Very often the woman will return to the abusive partner because she does not want to become a single parent; she feels responsible for her children and she feels they should stay with the father; she may get pressure from her family to return to her partner; she loves her partner and hopes that the violence will stop.

Most local authorities have set up a support network for women who have experienced violence. This network includes members of social services, the health team, the police and women's groups.

Throughout our lives we may experience neglect and lack of support that can have a serious effect on our personal development and our ability to form intimate relationships.

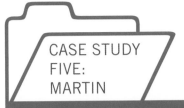

## CASE STUDY FIVE: MARTIN

Martin is 14. His parents are divorced. He lives with his mother. He never sees his father. His mother has had a lot of boyfriends in the last five years. She works full-time and is often out in the evenings and at weekends. She goes on holiday and leaves Martin on his own. There is never anything to eat in the house, so Martin has to buy food when his mother gives him money. Martin tries to keep the house looking tidy, and he does his own washing. He spends a lot of time on his own. Martin finds it difficult to make friends at school. He can't afford to go out with his class mates. Sometimes he helps out on a stall at the local market. Martin feels very depressed. He is behind with his studies. Sometimes he feels so depressed in the morning that he can't be bothered to go to school. He can't see any point in living, but he doesn't know who to talk to about how he feels.

## Discussion

Probably Martin's mother isn't aware of how he feels. Adolescence is an awkward time (see Chapter 2) and emotional support is a key factor in helping young people make the transition to adult life. The effects of lack of support can be seen in this case study. Suggest ways in which Martin could be supported.

Neglect and lack of support may occur at any time in one's life, but particularly in later life.

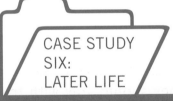

## CASE STUDY SIX: LATER LIFE

A practice nurse visited 37 older people aged over 75 as part of the over 75 health check that is required by the NHS. One of the remarks made by a patient was 'It is nice to be treated as a person and not just a number'. All the patients she saw said that the worst aspect of their lives was social isolation. Several were housebound, and only saw the district nurse or the milkman. Many of their families lived far away and phoned occasionally. These patients felt that social contact was very important, and the isolation they experienced affected how they saw themselves. Their self-esteem and their ability to relate to others were affected by the lack of social relationships.

# SELF-CONCEPT

All people have a view of themselves known as the self-concept. This is based upon the beliefs that they have of themselves as a person, and also on what other people think about them. Figure 4.23 shows the factors that affect a person's self-concept. We will look at these factors in turn.

## Age

In order for a concept of "self" to develop, you first have to see yourself as a separate physical being. This is established by the age of 15–18 months, when the toddler begins to understand that he or she is an individual. Parents and others tell the toddler he is a good boy or she is a pretty girl, and this is how children receive information about themselves. As we become older, we use information from others to confirm our view of ourselves. Our friends, partners and family all reinforce our opinion of ourselves. As well

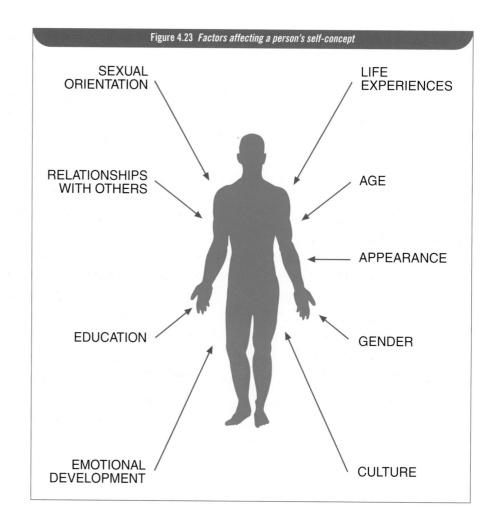

**Figure 4.23** *Factors affecting a person's self-concept*

SEXUAL ORIENTATION

LIFE EXPERIENCES

RELATIONSHIPS WITH OTHERS

AGE

APPEARANCE

EDUCATION

GENDER

EMOTIONAL DEVELOPMENT

CULTURE

as the information we receive from others, media images also reinforce our view of ourselves and the image we present to others.

Research has been done by Montmayer and Eisen (1977) to show how self-concept changes with age. In their study, 50 young people between the ages of 10 and 18 were asked to describe themselves in 20 statements. Younger boys and girls tended to describe themselves, giving their name, age and interests. Older people tended to give a more personal reply, mentioning their type of personality. Rosenberg (1979) interviewed children between the ages of 8 and 18 and grouped their responses into four main areas: physical, character, relationships and inner self.

Rosenberg concluded that younger children's responses were based on physical factors, but older children were more aware of character traits and inner qualities.

# Activity

Below are two examples of responses given in a more recent study done by a college student.

**Jodie, aged 11**

I am 11 years old, I have one brother and one sister, I have fair hair and blue eyes. I play with my friends in the park. I used to live in London. Now I live in Norfolk. I like art at school but I hate maths. I have a cat and a dog. I have a bedroom of my own. I have a bike.

**Beverley, aged 15**

I am 15 years old. I am a daughter and a sister. I have a good personality. I love going to the gym and dancing. When I leave school I want to be an air hostess. On Saturdays I like to hang around with my friends. I think I am a kind person. I cry in sad films. I am doing my GCSEs. I love my gran.

1.  What are the main differences between the two responses?
    You could draw up columns for **physical**, **character traits**, **relationships**, and **inner qualities** (see Figure 4.24) write the responses down and tick the column.
    We can see that the younger girl has more responses in the physical column – her age, where she lives, what she looks like, while the older girl talks about her friends, her personality and her feelings.
2.  You could do this experiment yourself, using young people of different ages. Don't forget to get permission from parents if you choose to ask a young child.

**Figure 4.24** *Category Analysis Form*

| P | C | R | I | PARTICIPANT Jodie<br>AGE 11                                       SEX. F |
|---|---|---|---|---|
| ✓ |   |   |   | I am eleven years old |
|   |   | ✓ |   | I have one brother and one sister |
| ✓ |   |   |   | I have fair hair and blue eyes |
| ✓ |   |   |   | I play with my friends in the park |
| ✓ |   |   |   | I used to live in London, now I live in Norfolk |
|   | ✓ |   |   | I like art at school |
|   | ✓ |   |   | I hate Maths |
| ✓ |   |   |   | I have a cat and a dog |
| ✓ |   |   |   | I have a bedroom of my own |
| ✓ |   |   |   | I have a bike |
|   |   |   |   |  |
| 7 | 2 | 1 | 0 | Column Totals                  Overall Total = 10 |

# Appearance

As we have said before, we are influenced in our self-concept by the opinion of others and by how we compare ourselves with **media images**. People tend to be more sensitive to this influence on their self-concept in their adolescence and adult lives. If you look at magazines or papers you can see that certain images of men and women are promoted. Women are supposed to be slim, well dressed and use make-up. Men are supposed to have athletic bodies and be well groomed. Role models such as Britney Spears or David Beckham show the aspirations of many young people. As we get older, appearance becomes less important. This could be because of other changes in our lives, such as parenthood, family commitments or more self-confidence in our feelings about ourselves. Experiments have been carried out where people have changed their appearance and they noticed a change in the way other people reacted to them – this showed how other people's reactions affect our self-image. One actress wore a 'fat suit' and found that people's attitudes were hostile and unfriendly. Another actress made herself up to look like an old woman and found that shop assistants ignored her in shops, and people generally tended to avoid responding to her. A white actor made his skin darker and changed his style of dress, more casual and 'hip hop', and found that white youths were aggressive to him. A student on a psychology course decided to test how helpful people would be to him if he was in a wheelchair in a busy shopping area. He found he was ignored or any comments were made to his friend who was pushing the wheelchair.

We can see from these examples that appearance can make a difference to the reactions of others to you, and in turn this can affect your self-concept.

# Gender

When a baby is born, it is biologically identified as either male (having a penis) or female (having a vagina). Gender refers to the psychological or social aspects we develop as we grow up. Gender identity is a clear understanding of ourselves as either male or female, and as part of our development we take on the expected social roles of males and females in our society. Boys play with action figures and are boisterous in play. Girls enjoy playing with dolls and are quieter. These are the **gender stereotypes** that we are expected to conform to.

Children know whether they are boys or girls by the age of two. Their play and choice of friends reflects their gender identity. Between the ages of three and five, boys and girls prefer to play with the same sex. By the ages of seven or eight the gender stereotypes for both girls and boys begin to weaken. Gender identity is reinforced through the media. Television adverts show traditional toys for boys and girls in the period before Christmas. Parents are also influential in promoting gender differences.

Expectations of others based on gender, can lead to problems if girls want to follow non-traditional female jobs, such as becoming car mechanics or plumbers. It can also be difficult for boys who want to be nurses or carers of family members. Ann Oakley did some studies when she interviewed housewives (*Housewife*, 1974). She was interested in the women's self-image and she asked them to answer the question 'Who am I?' ten times. One of the women replied as follows:

I am a housewife.

I am going to the shop.

I am a mother.

I am a good housewife.

I am a mother of four children.

I am a wife.

I am a good cleaner.

I am a good washer.

I am always working.

This woman was a full-time housewife. Do you think women who are mothers today would reply in the same way? (the study was done between 1969 and 1970).

## Culture

Culture is related to our systems of beliefs, practices, dress, language, and religious beliefs, which all influence our lives.

For example, some cultures do not approve of the use of alcohol, and have strict rules about marriage and some aspects of family life.

Culture, especially ethnic identity, affects our self-concept by influencing our feelings of belonging and our ideas about membership of different social groups.

Culture and ethnic identity give us a sense of shared values. This is an important part of socialisation of children and setting standards of behaviour. Different cultural groups may experience discrimination and this will have an effect on self-concept.

## Emotional development

Emotional development occurs throughout the life cycle, and is affected by the experiences we have at different times during our lives. Emotional development is linked to becoming a confident and secure adult with high self-esteem. Research shows that children who have had a secure and stable relationship with a parent have higher self-esteem, whereas children who have had an insecure and unstable background show more tantrums and aggression, and this experience will affect them in adult relationships in later life.

---

**CASE STUDY FIVE: CULTURE**

Two black parents have decided to keep their three children away from school, because they believe they have been treated unfairly. What effect could this action have on the self-concept of a, the parents and b, the children?

---

# Education

Education can affect your self-concept. If teachers tells you you are lazy or not very clever, this will have an effect on the way you see yourself – you may accept what they say and this could have a negative effect on your self-image and your performance at school. On the other hand, if teachers praise you and tell you that you will succeed, this will give you a positive self-image and high self-esteem.

**Labelling** is the term used by psychologists when they talk about how people are labelled in a particular way by people who have power (teachers, employers, parents). If the label is accepted by the child or person, then it becomes part of their view of themselves.

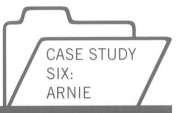

CASE STUDY
SIX:
ARNIE

When Arnie went to infants school, he used to enjoy playing with a friend and getting up to mischief. Once they flooded the washroom area by leaving the taps on. When Arnie's parents came to the parents' evening they were told Arnie was a naughty boy. Arnie became so used to everyone saying he was a naughty boy that after a while his behaviour reflected the label. Everyone, including the other children, expected him to be naughty. Psychologists talk about the '**self-fullfiling prophecy**', which means that after a while behaviour develops according to the expectations of people. Because everyone expected Arnie to be naughty, he continued to behave in a naughty way.

Figure 4.25 shows how this can work.

Being naughty can increase your status with other children, but it also affects how you see yourself.

The example of Arnie shows how education can affect your self-image. If you are seen to be successful, then this will give you high self-esteem and a positive self-image. If you have a negative experience, this can make you feel less capable and unsure of your ability.

# Relationships with others

As we have already seen, relationships with other people are very important throughout our lives. Friends can make us feel supported and happy about ourselves. However, if relationships break down or we feel people are behaving badly towards us this can affect our self-image.

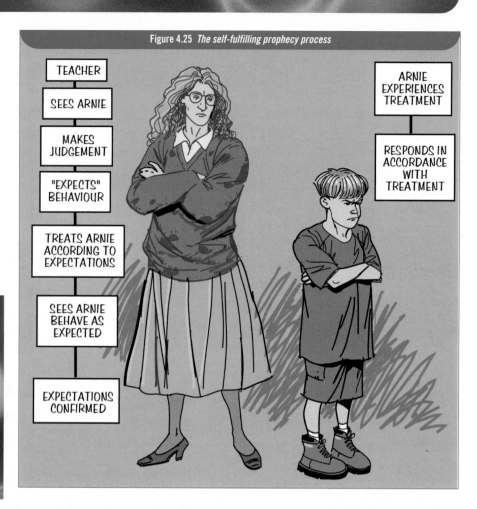
Figure 4.25 *The self-fulfilling prophecy process*

TEACHER

SEES ARNIE

MAKES JUDGEMENT

"EXPECTS" BEHAVIOUR

TREATS ARNIE ACCORDING TO EXPECTATIONS

SEES ARNIE BEHAVE AS EXPECTED

EXPECTATIONS CONFIRMED

ARNIE EXPERIENCES TREATMENT

RESPONDS IN ACCORDANCE WITH TREATMENT

## Activity

Look at the following case studies and think how you might support the people who are having problems with their relationships.

## CASE STUDY ONE: JATINDER

Jatinder (who is 24) has recently started a new job in a health centre where she is working as a receptionist. Most of the other women there are older than her, but they all seem to be quite pleasant apart from Sue, the Practice Manager. Sue is in her 40s and Jatinder feels that she is always criticising what she is doing and picking on her. It has got to the point when Jatinder dreads going into work. One afternoon when a baby clinic was taking place, Jatinder was talking to one of the mothers and telling her about where to find information about child care; Sue came over to her and interrupted, saying that it wasn't her business to give that kind of information. Jatinder burst into tears. Later, when she was at home, she told her mother that she couldn't cope with the job any more, she was useless and no-one would want to employ her.

## CASE STUDY TWO: FRANCINE

Francine is 15 and working for her GCSEs. Francine has an older sister who got pregnant when she was 14, had the baby and left home to live with her boyfriend's family. Francine's parents are very anxious about her and don't want her to go out with boys or stay out late at night. Francine feels they don't trust her, and after a while she begins to tell them lies about where she is going and what she is doing. Francine has met a boy, Robert, whom she likes very much. She decides to go out with him one Saturday evening and tells her parents she is going to see her friend Maria. When Francine gets back home, she finds her parents are furious with her. They phoned Maria who told them Francine was not with her. Francine's parents are threatening to keep her in the house all the time when she isn't at school.

## CASE STUDY THREE: SHELIA

Sheila has been married to Mike for 20 years and they have three teenage children. Sheila recently went back to work. Paul, one of the men in the office, asked her out for a drink. Sheila went with him. He paid her a lot of attention and said how attractive she was. This made Sheila feel wonderful, as her husband worked long hours and never told her he loved her or took her out. Sheila started to go regularly to the pub; she bought herself new clothes and lost weight, but her husband didn't seem to notice. There was a weekend training session arranged for Sheila's department, that included an overnight stay in a hotel. Sheila went on this and during the weekend she spent the night with Paul. When she next saw Paul, he was busy talking to a new girl who had joined the staff and he ignored her. 'I see Paul is lining up his next conquest', said Anne, who worked with Sheila. Sheila suddenly realised that what she thought had been a possible serious relationship had been a 'bit of fun' for Paul.

## Sexual orientation

This is a term used in **sociology** to describe the focus of an individual's sex drive. **Heterosexual** orientation is when a person is attracted to the opposite sex. **Homosexual** orientation is attraction towards the same sex – gay men and lesbian women. Homosexual activity was seen to be illegal in the UK until *The Sexual Offences Act* of 1967, when homosexual acts between men over the age of 21 were allowed. In 1993 MPs voted to lower the age of consent for homosexual men from 21 to 18. In 1998, the House of Commons voted in favour of lowering the consent for homosexuals to 16 (the same as for heterosexuals) but the House of Lords blocked this legislation .

**Homophobia** means hatred and fear of homosexuals. This fear can result in bullying and physical attacks on lesbian and gay people. Many people who have realised that they are homosexual, began to be aware of this when they were 14 or younger. As we have already seen, adolescence can be a very difficult time for a young person, and coping with the idea that he or she may also be homosexual is an additional stress factor. For boys in particular, heterosexuality is seen to be part of masculinity, and part of the male identity. Boys can be under a great deal of pressure from their friends and family to adopt typical male behaviour – liking football, drinking and other pursuits seen as "masculine". Girls are sometimes described as being 'tomboys' if they tend to be interested in sport and less interested in make-up and clothes. Media images of young people in pop and teen magazines tend to focus on the stereotype of feminine girls and masculine boys. For a young person coming to terms with their homosexuality, these pressures can affect their self-concept. They are also concerned about how their parents and friends will react if they try to explain how they feel. Feeling different from others may lead to feelings of isolation and lack of self-worth, which will make the young person feel depressed, anxious and lonely.

# THE EFFECTS OF LIFE EVENTS ON PERSONAL DEVELOPMENT

Life experiences can have a positive or negative effect on our self-concept. We have already looked at some life experiences, such as the experience of school and work. Life experiences can be on a very personal and individual level, such as our experience of family life, but they can also be on a larger scale when many people are affected. In the Second World War many children were evacuated to the country and separated from their parents. Men went into the armed forces and women worked in a variety of jobs, including working in factories making a contribution to the war effort.

We can see that some life experiences are shared with others and others are very personal.

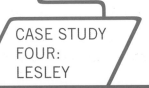

## CASE STUDY FOUR: LESLEY

Lesley was five at the beginning of World War 2. She had a sister of eight. They lived in London with their parents. When war was declared, Lesley and her sister were evacuated (with the whole school and their teachers) to Cornwall. Lesley's mother stayed in London and her father was working for the War Office. Lesley saw her mother occasionally, but it was not until the war ended when she was 10 that she went back to live with her mother. Lesley and her sister were looked after by a farmer and his wife during the war. They were expected to help in the farm. They found life in the country very strange – they had never seen cows or other farm animals before. Although the farmer and his wife were quite kind, Lesley really missed her parents. Even now, Lesley talks about the war as being a very difficult time. She felt she missed out on her childhood. Because of shortages, Lesley had few toys or sweets. She felt that her parents could have kept her with them as she was so young, and she still feels that her parents couldn't have loved her if they allowed her to be evacuated. When she moved back to live with them she never felt settled.

Many people experienced these changes. These were life experiences that affected many people.

**Self-concept has several components:**

- **Self-image** – how you see yourself and what you know about yourself. This is affected according to your cultural background. In most Western societies, people tend to focus on their individual personality traits. In Japanese and other cultures, people tend to describe themselves as part of a social group.
- **Ideal self** – refers to the person you would like to be. We can be influenced by the media, parents and teachers.
- **Self-esteem** – refers to how you feel about yourself and judge yourself. How much do we like the kind of person we are? Do we accept ourselves as we are?

Self-esteem is shaped by a number of factors:

- comparison of self-image and the ideal self we would like to be
- information we receive from others about ourselves
- social identity – the group we belong to.

# Activity

This is an exercise that has often been used in college and work groups to improve the members self-esteem. It is best done in groups of between six and eight people. Everyone in the group has to think of a positive thing to say about each member of the group and say it to them. This is quite a good exercise to do at the end of a course or at the end of a training session. We all need to think about supporting others, especially if we are working in health and social care, where many of the client groups have low self-esteem.

One way we assess or evaluate ourselves is to compare our self-image with our ideal self; the closer we feel our self-image is to our ideal self, the higher our self-esteem is.

On page 310, Danielle said that in her work with families she found that all the mothers who were having problems suffered from low self-esteem. Perhaps they had compared their self-image as a mother to the ideal self of what they felt a perfect mother would be like, and because there was a gap between the two, this had an effect on their self-esteem. We can see plenty of examples of this at school, work and in family life, where people feel they don't measure up to the ideal and this results in low self-esteem.

We all need to concentrate on how we can develop our self-esteem and see ourselves in a good light, and perhaps avoid situations that reduce our self-esteem.

Life events are expected or unexpected experiences that can have a major impact on an individual's personal development.

# Relationship changes

## Predictable events

### Marriage

In 2002 marriage rates are increasing. Marriage is a life event that is celebrated by many people each year. Marriage involves a major change in personal development, especially a first marriage. The role of the married couple changes. Instead of being part of their birth families they are now separate from their parents, and their main emotional and psychological commitment is to each other. As well as changing the relationship between the parents and the new couple, new relationships are also formed between the in-laws who become part of the wider family network. In some cases the married couple may have to move away from their parents because of work or housing, and this will make the couple very dependent on each other for support.

### Living with a partner

As we have already seen on page 324–325, many people are choosing to live with someone rather than get married. Some people live together before they get married, so we can see living together as a

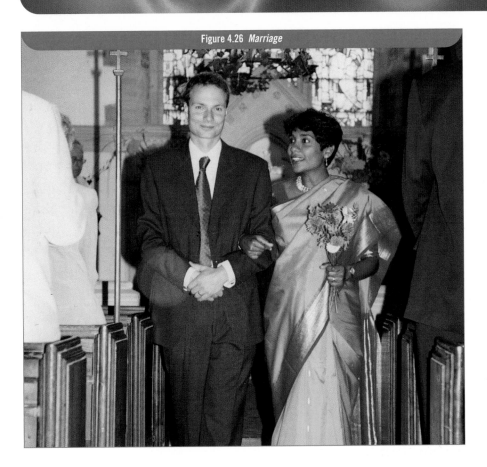

Figure 4.26 *Marriage*

predictable event. Because there is usually no formal legal arrangement between couples who live together, this may cause stress on the couple, especially if they then go on to have children. Family members may disapprove of what they see as 'living in sin'. The couple themselves may see the arrangement as temporary, and this may lead to feelings of insecurity. Although many people live together very happily and see marriage as 'a piece of paper they don't need', other people may feel that if their partner is unwilling to make a commitment of marriage to them, they are not important to them, and this can lead to feelings of low self-esteem. Because they don't feel secure in the relationship, they can't relax and this affects their personal development.

### Having children

Although the birth rate is reducing in the UK, many people still expect to have children, whether they are married or not. Parenthood involves a major change in a person's life, with the additional pressures of responsibility and money worries. It is

# Activity

Karl and Charlotte have been going out together for three years, since they met when they were in the Sixth Form. Both their families approve of the relationship, but Charlotte's mother keeps making remarks like, 'the neighbours are wondering when you are going to get wed', and 'Your Gran thinks it's time Karl made an honest woman of you'. Unknown to their families, Karl and Charlotte have been looking at flats in their area, as they are thinking of renting a place together. Charlotte is nearing the end of her nursing training, and Karl has been offered promotion in the council, where he works in the housing department. They both feel they don't want to have children for a while – Charlotte is on the pill, and they are not sure about getting married as they are still only 21. They want to live together and see how it works out, but they are dreading telling their parents.

Imagine you are a friend of theirs. How would you put forward arguments for and against them living together, rather than getting married?

often said that once a couple become parents, they become adults. Although many people find having a child a wonderful experience, it can also be very demanding, especially for the woman. In spite of ideas about the 'new man', most women find they take on the main responsibility for child care.

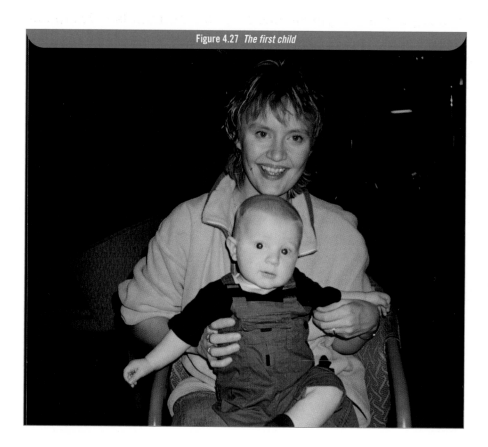

Figure 4.27 *The first child*

Parents also need to decide on how to bring up the child; whether both parents can continue to work; how child care can be arranged. Other family members may also be involved, especially-grandparents who may give conflicting advice, or criticise how child care is being managed.

Parenthood is often described as a 24-hour-a-day, 365-days-a-year job, with no time off, no pay and little recognition. Mothers may find it difficult to make the change from going to work, going out socially and doing things on the spur of the moment, to looking after a demanding baby, a reduced social life and less money to spend. If the mother had a difficult pregnancy and birth, she may also feel that she has lost her figure; that no-one, including her husband, will find her attractive any more, and that staying at home affects her self-confidence. Lack of sleep may affect her energy levels and she may be depressed.

Although having a baby can be a positive, enjoyable experience which can make a woman feel fulfilled, it can also feel rather a burden for both partners. The father may feel that all his partner's attention is focused on the baby and that he is ignored, so this can affect his self-image.

### *Birth of sibling*

Although more people are deciding to limit their families to one child, in the past people tended to have larger families, partly because of lack of effective contraception. Sometimes children are close together in age, but sometimes there is a gap of several years. When a new baby is born, it can be difficult for a child who is used to having a lot of attention. Sibling jealousy often results in very demanding behaviour for some time, until the family adjusts to the new social relationships. Recent research suggests that the older child needs to feel that they are being treated in exactly the same way as the new baby. Children can feel jealous and anxious about the arrival of a new baby. It is important to allow the child to express their feelings, perhaps by active play and taking out their aggression on a soft toy. Sibling rivalry can continue throughout childhood and into adulthood. This can be caused by one child feeling that their sibling is favoured by their parents, and these feelings can affect personal development as, when they become an adult, they can still feel rejected and inadequate in their relationships.

### Death of a friend or relative

Although we know that we will all die, death can still have a great impact on our personal development. We expect older relatives to die before we do, and we know that we are likely to see the deaths of our parents and grandparents. In the UK, death is still seen as a subject many people prefer not to talk about, although death is marked by funeral services and rituals when the person's life is celebrated. Death of an older family member can be seen as a release, especially if they have been ill for a long time, but the death of this person can leave a gap in the lives of the people who are left. It is natural to feel sad and to miss the person.

Research has shown that if there was a good relationship between the person who died and the bereaved person, then sadness will gradually be replaced with acceptance, and the good memories of the past. If there was a difficult relationship, the person left may feel guilty and find it difficult to get over the death. In this case professional help may be needed. When our older family members die, we then take on the roles of leading the family. For example, in *Eastenders*, when Pauline Fowler's mother died, Pauline took over the role as the dominant female in the family.

## Unexpected events

### Divorce

When a couple meet, fall in love and get married, they decide they are going to stay together for the rest of their lives and make vows to that effect. They do not intend to get divorced. The breakdown of the marriage and the process of divorce have an emotional impact on the couple. When the couple have children, these problems are increased, as decisions will have to be made about who will have care of the children. Separate accommodation and income arrangements will have to be made. Dealing with solicitors and courts can also be stressful. The grandparents will also be affected. If the couple find new partners, this will bring in other relationships. Both men and women can feel guilty and have a sense of failure over the ending of the marriage. The woman may have to make major adjustments to her life, if she has to work full-time to support the family, taking responsibility for money and running a household that she had previously left to her husband, or shared in the past. Divorce can be seen as a challenge, and some women find it a positive challenge and develop their confidence and ability to hold down a job. Others may feel rejected by their husbands. They feel they will never find another partner and feel lonely and depressed. Research has shown that divorced men are more likely to remarry, but that second marriages are more likely to fail. Divorced men are more likely to become ill, and turn to alcohol and other forms of addiction. Figure 4.28 shows the divorce and remarriage rates. Identify the main patterns you see.

### Unexpected death

Although we may expect our older family members to die, accidental or sudden deaths can cause additional problems. This is especially the case with the deaths of children and babies. Parents feel guilty and ashamed. Their distress can put a great strain on the marriage (see Case Study 5). The FSID (Foundation for the Study of Infant Deaths)

is an organisation that provides support for parents who have lost a child through cot death.

Luckily, Stella and John had support, but we can see from this case study that unexpected deaths can have a serious impact on our personal development, affecting our self-confidence and our ability to make relationships.

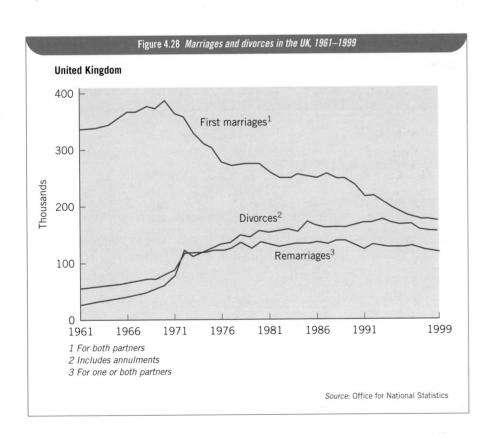

Figure 4.28 *Marriages and divorces in the UK, 1961–1999*

1 For both partners
2 Includes annulments
3 For one or both partners

Source: Office for National Statistics

## CASE STUDY FIVE:

John and Stella were expecting their first baby. They were very excited about it. They moved to a new house two months before the baby was due, in a new area so they did not know anyone, but they registered with a GP in the area and Stella was booked into the local hospital. Stella had a long and difficult delivery. She had a little girl. Because of concerns about the baby, it wasn't until the baby was a week old that Stella came home. The baby cried all the time, and Stella was very tired and was having difficulty feeding the baby. The health visitor advised Stella to change to bottle feeding. After three weeks the baby was settling down and was sleeping through the night. When she was six weeks old, John went into the baby's room early in the morning. The baby was white and not breathing. John tried to revive the baby while Stella called for an ambulance. When they got to the hospital they were told the baby had died from a cot death. They couldn't believe that the baby was dead. The christening had been booked for the next day and they had to tell everyone what had happened.

John and Stella felt they had done something wrong to make the baby die, although the doctor told them that the death was from natural causes. They had to attend an inquest, but before this happened they were interviewed by the police. The case was reported in the local paper, which they found very upsetting. The GP contacted a befriender who visited the family and listened to them.

They were nervous of having another baby, they felt they did not deserve to have children; they also felt angry that their baby had died. After several years they had three more children, but they still remember Helen and visit her grave often.

# Physical Changes

## Expected changes

### *Puberty*

Adolescence and puberty can be disturbing times. Both girls and boys can develop secondary sexual characteristics at different times. It can be difficult for a 15-year-old boy who is shorter than the rest of his class mates, or for a girl who started her periods in junior school and found there were no facilities for the disposal of sanitary protection. The development of breasts or the lack of them can cause feelings of inadequacy and lack of self-confidence. Spots, braces on the teeth, and sudden growth spurts can all be disturbing and confusing. It is important that the young person is given positive support and reassurance during this time. As we

Figure 4.29 *A Foundation for the Study of Infant Death leaflet*

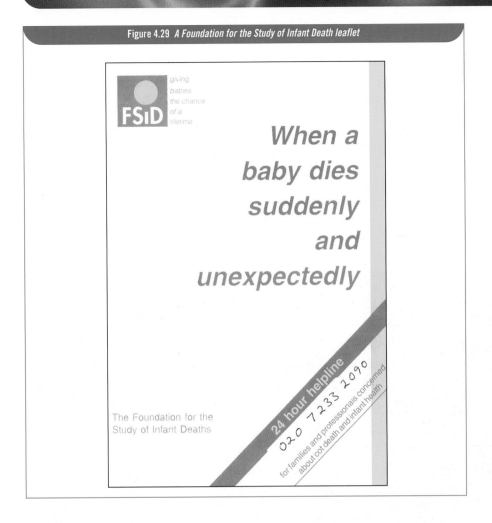

have seen in Chapter 2, adolescence is a difficult stage between childhood and adulthood. It is important that young people feel valued and respected so that they have a positive self-concept. This provides a firm basis for adjustment to adult life.

### The menopause

Just as puberty is an expected change, so is the menopause. This marks the end of a woman's reproductive life phase, and can be seen as a positive change as it means that anxiety about unwanted pregnancy is removed. It can also be seen as a negative time, when a woman may feel physically unattractive as her hormones change, and some of the physical symptoms can be unpleasant – night sweats, increased anxiety, dry skin and headaches. Although the GP can prescribe effective medication to assist the physical changes, it is important that the woman maintains a positive self-image. Her children may be older and she may have more time for herself and her husband. She may be able to take up interests she never had time to do before.

## Unexpected changes

### *Accident or illness leading to disability*

Some people are born or inherit physical or learning disabilities. Others acquire a disability as a result of accident or illness, for example being involved in a car accident. People who become disabled have to adapt their lifestyle to cope with the disability.

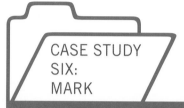

CASE STUDY
SIX:
MARK

**Mark's story.**

Mark is now 35.

'I was 28 and I had just got married. I used to play rugby on Saturdays. Some days I noticed I was seeing double, but I put it down to overdoing things and getting tired. I then started getting pins and needles in my arm and leg on the left side. One day I got out of bed and nearly fell over, my balance seemed to go. I went to see the GP. He referred me to the specialist. After a lot of tests I was told I had MS (multiple sclerosis). I was absolutely gutted. I had just got a new job teaching in a school in the West Country, and we had been thinking about starting a family. The head teacher was really helpful, but my wife found it all too much and we split up soon after I was diagnosed – probably my fault as I became very sorry for myself and difficult to live with.

Since I was diagnosed I have had some flare ups when I can hardly move and I have been in hospital for assessment. My car has been adapted so I don't need to use the foot pedals. I have moved into a ground-floor flat. I am still working full time at the moment. I can get about the school using a stick, but I might need to use a wheelchair at some point.

The worst thing about the disease is that you don't know how fast it will progress. I might be like I am at the moment for a while. I look at rugby on the television and I really miss playing. I have found the adjustment has been really difficult, as I was so fit and independent. I have a new girl friend now, and that has made a tremendous difference. If anything I feel the experience of MS has made me more aware of the importance of enjoying life while I can and making the most of every day. I couldn't have coped without my friends.'

We can see from Mark's story that even very negative events can be a means to achieve personal growth. Not everyone may have Mark's resilience, and adapting to serious illness and disability can be a challenge.

# Changes in life circumstances

## Expected

### Starting school

This is one of the first predictable life events for all children. Beginning **primary school** is a turning point in children's lives. It means that the child is going to leave the support of parents and the home setting, and move into the wider social setting of school, where new patterns of behaviour will occur. Many children (and their parents) find the first day of school very frightening. Many schools recognise this and have a system where children start off with a half day and then move to a full day at school. With more nursery classes attached to primary schools, children become used to the school. The move to **secondary school** can be more difficult, especially if the child has not managed to get into the school preferred by their parents. Children need the support of parents, brothers and sisters, and teachers to cope successfully with this life change.

### Starting work

Starting work represents the transition from childhood to adulthood. Starting work means that we have to be responsible, and behave as independent adults. However, although work can be exciting and stimulating, it can also be boring. All jobs can be repetitive. As part of our personal development we need to be able to adapt to the demands made on us by work. We develop skills, such as time management and attention to detail, that may be very important. We also need to develop social skills, as in most jobs we will be working with people as colleagues or as clients.

In Chapter 2 we looked at the skills needed in jobs in health and social care. The development of these skills is all part of our personal development.

### Retirement

Although we may spend much of our life in work, the time spent in retirement is increasing as we live longer. Some people see retirement as a release from the daily grind and routine of work, but some people see retirement as a time of anxiety. They feel they have lost their identity, especially if their job was very important to them and had high status. Women who have spent time bringing up a family may worry that they will not have enough money to manage, as they may not have much in the way of a pension. We still have to eat, maintain a house or flat, keep warm and pay the bills when we retire, even though we are not working. Many retired people miss the social contact that they had at work. As we have already seen on page 246, most people over 75 visited by a practice nurse felt social isolation was the main problem they faced.

If retirement can be a time to do those things that were not possible when we were working, then this helps personal development, but if people experience poverty and loneliness, this has a very negative effect on people's self-image.

## Unexpected changes

### *Redundancy*

Redundancy happens when an employer decides that a job no longer exists and the worker is given notice of redundancy, losing their job through no fault of their own. This can happen when two firms merge, or there is an economic recession. Redundancy can have a great effect on an individual's self-esteem, as well as affecting their income. People who have been made redundant can feel worthless, especially if they have been in the company for many years and worked hard. They can wonder what the point was of all the years they spent working, if they are then told they have to

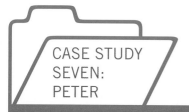

CASE STUDY
SEVEN:
PETER

**Peter's story**

I had worked for the company for 17 years in their office in the City. There had been a lot of changes when we were taken over by another firm, but redundancy had never been mentioned. I went into the office as usual on the Monday and was called into the manager's office. I was told that changes were being made and that new I.T. systems were being introduced. They felt that as I was 50 I would find it difficult to cope with the changes and my old job would not exist any more. I was asked to clear my desk and be out of the office by lunchtime. I felt really ill, I couldn't believe what was happening. I had worked really hard for the firm for all those years. I was worried about the family – we had four children, and three were still at school. My wife worked part time. I went home and went to bed I felt so awful. I had to tell my wife when she got in from work. I had made a lot of friends in the firm and in the City, but when I rang them they didn't want to talk to me. They said they would look out for a job for me, but they never rang me back. I wrote 60 letters to people I knew asking for a job, but I wasn't successful. In the end, I found another job at a smaller company on lower pay, but I shall never feel secure again. You never know it might happen again.

leave. In some cases, the decision to make workers redundant can happen overnight.

We can see from Peter's story (Case Study 7) that redundancy can have a severe and lasting effect on someone's self-image.

In this section we have looked at some examples of expected and unexpected life events that may have a serious effect on an individual's personal development. In some cases friends and family can offer support, but sometimes support may be needed from other people if the event leads to illness such as depression, or the individual is on their own, or the problem is something that the individual can't discuss with friends or family.

## Professional support

GPs are reporting an increase in advising patients who have social problems rather than medical problems. A patient may see the GP because they are not sleeping, but by talking to the patient the GP realises that the problem is to do with work, family situations or other difficulties. Most surgeries can now refer patients to a counsellor who will see the patient for about six sessions. On the NHS, this service is free, but patients can also refer themselves to private counsellors, when they would have to pay.

As we have seen in Chapter 2, there are many professionals who can help with family problems related to child care. The health visitor can offer advice and support. Social workers can also offer support in a range of problems, especially related to illness, disability, poverty and unemployment.

## Voluntary and other services that offer support

There are many charities and organisations that offer support. We have already discussed the support given by FSID to bereaved parents. The charity **Cruse** can offer support to bereaved people; the **Citizens Advice Bureau** can give advice on people's rights and benefits; **Age Concern** can offer support to older people; **Relate** offers support for people who are having problems with their marriage or partnerships. Local churches and religious groups can also offer support and guidance.

Many of the professional and voluntary groups that offer support will be listed in local directories or in the library. The Internet also gives details of organisations that give support to particular groups. Organisations such as RNID (the Royal Institute for the Deaf) and the RNIB (the Royal Institute for the Blind) offer support to disabled people and have a website.

Self-help groups are a further source of support. **No Panic** is a self-help group that was set up to support people who experience panic attacks. Panic attacks can occur following life changes, and finding support from a local group can be very helpful. You can find a full list of self-help groups on the following web site www.self-help.org.uk.

## Activity

Look at the following examples of life changes and think of at least two types of support you might use if you were in this situation:

▶ break up of a marriage or long-term relationship
▶ becoming visually impaired
▶ the death of a close friend
▶ being diagnosed with a serious illness
▶ the birth of your first child
▶ starting your nursing training
▶ getting into serious debt
▶ leaving home and starting college
▶ losing your job.

As we can see, we may all experience difficulties during our lives. Expected and unexpected events may force us to cope with change. Our reactions to these events can affect our health and well-being, so it is important that we find ways to cope. If we are unable to adjust to changes, this may result in serious physical, psychological and social problems which will affect our self-image and our health.

# REFERENCES

Rosenberg, M. (1979) *Conceiving the Self*. New York, Basic Books.

Thomson et al (2000) *Health and Social Care Vocational A Level*. London, Hodder and Stoughton.

Thomson et al (2000) *Health and Social Care Intermediate GNVQ*. London, Hodder and Stoughton.

Woods, B. (2000) *Basics in Psychology, Second Edition*. London, Hodder and Stoughton.

# USEFUL ADDRESSES

If you contact a charity it is helpful to enclose postage stamps. Many charities have their own websites and this may be a quicker way of obtaining information.

### Homestart
2, Salisbury Road
Leicester LE1 7QR
www.home-start.org.uk

### FSID (Foundation for the Study of Infant Deaths)
Artillery House
London SW1P 1RT
www.sids.org.uk/fsid

### No Panic
93, Brands Farm Way
Telford TF3 2JQ

### Cruse Bereavement Care
126, Sheen Road,
Richmond
Surrey TW9 1UR

### Relate (relationship problems)
Herbert Gray College
Little Church Street
Rugby CV21 3AP
www.relate.org.uk

### RNID
www.rnid.org.uk

### RNIB
www.rnib.org.uk

### Answers
p. 278: 6 months

# Index

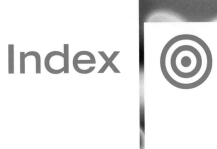